SCIENCE AND BABIES

Private Decisions,
Public Dilemmas

Suzanne Wymelenberg
for the
INSTITUTE OF MEDICINE

NATIONAL ACADEMY PRESS
Washington, DC   1990

National Academy Press ● 2101 Constitution Avenue, N.W. ● Washington, D.C. 20418

This publication is based on presentations at the annual meeting of the Institute of Medicine held in Washington, D.C., on October 19, 1988. The views expressed are those of the participants and do not necessarily reflect those of the Institute of Medicine.

The Institute of Medicine was chartered in 1970 by the National Academy of Sciences to enlist distinguished members of appropriate professions in the examination of policy matters pertaining to the health of the public. In this, the Institute acts both under the Academy's 1863 congressional charter responsibility to be an adviser to the federal government and its own initiative in identifying issues of medical care, research, and education.

This project was supported by a grant from the R. W. Johnson Pharmaceutical Research Institute, formed in a recent reorganization of the research and development divisions of Ortho Pharmaceutical Corp., Ortho Biotech, McNeil Pharmaceutical, and Cilag International.

Library of Congress Cataloging-in-Publication Data

Wymelenberg, Suzanne.
    Science and babies : private decisions, public dilemmas / Suzanne
Wymelenberg.
        p.   cm.
    Includes bibliographical references.
    ISBN 0-309-04140-6.—ISBN 0-309-04136-8 (pbk.)
    1. Human reproduction—Social aspects. 2. Contraception—Social
aspects. 3. Teenage pregnancy—Social aspects. 4. Human
reproductive technology—Moral and ethical aspects. I. Title.
RG133.W96   1990   90-35111
176—dc20   CIP

Printed in the United States of America

Preface

Discussion of personal reproductive health is generally reserved for the most private of settings: between partners, or between health provider and patient. Yet in the past decade, new developments in reproductive science and ongoing political conflict have increasingly thrust matters of conception and contraception squarely into the public spotlight.

At its Annual Meeting, October 19-20, 1988, the Institute of Medicine devoted a daylong symposium to "Advances in Reproductive Biology: Implications for Research, Application, and Policy Development." This book, authored by Suzanne Wymelenberg, draws on that meeting of experts. It describes the state of our understanding of human fertility and allied issues, such as teenage pregnancy and prenatal care. It is clear throughout that both evolutionary and revolutionary advances in reproductive research lie ahead.

The book concludes with chapters highlighting ethical concerns raised by interventions in human reproduction and public policy issues—difficult choices—that America faces in the 1990s. Forthright public discussion of sexual topics usually confined to private conversations will be necessary, if exciting gains in our understanding of reproductive biology are to be sensibly translated into gains in reproductive health. This book is directed toward energizing that process.

SAMUEL O. THIER
President
Institute of Medicine

Contents

SCIENCE AND BABIES

Private Decisions,
Public Dilemmas

1

Reproductive Health Issues

Reproductive health, ideally, means that every baby is wanted and planned for and that every pregnant woman has access to the resources she needs for her own and her baby's robustness. It means putting more effort into improving the survival, health, and development of infants. It also means helping to solve problems of infertility for men and women who want to have a baby and cannot. It means finding more acceptable, safer contraceptive methods and making existing methods more available, with vigorous dissemination of information about contraception and other health matters that affect reproduction. It means increasing support to eliminate or alleviate genetic diseases. Most important, it means developing the view that healthy reproduction is intrinsic to the vitality of the nation and, with it, the commitment to use all possible means, including education, research, ethical inquiry, and political action, to achieve that goal.

Since 1980 the reproductive health status of Americans has deteriorated. The rates for unintended pregnancy and abortion in the United States are among the highest in the Western world, and our rates for adolescent pregnancy, abortion, and childbearing are the highest. In infant mortality, a key indicator of national health, the United States ranks twentieth among industrialized nations, behind Hong Kong and Singapore. Despite our considerable research resources, American women have fewer contraceptive choices than their European counterparts. More than half the 6 million pregnancies that occur annually in this country are unintended, and half those unintended pregnancies—about 1.6 million—end in abortion. Meanwhile, concern about infertility appears to be increasing among many women and men.

The United States has long been a leader in clinical obstetrics and pediatrics. U.S. professionals launched the "contraceptive revolution" in the 1960s with the development of the pill and the modern IUD. Yet reproductive health in this country has deteriorated in recent years as changes in society and biology have collided. Today, most young women and men are not prepared to take on adult responsibilities until they are in their 20s, but their bodies often are sexually mature by age 12. Sexual development brings the risk of pregnancy and sexually transmitted diseases. The arrival of puberty before social maturity causes problems for which few answers exist. Fearful of arousing protests from religious groups and antiabortionists, government does little to support contraceptive development and sex education. There is great reluctance to advertise contraceptives, although the alternative has been a very high abortion rate and increased welfare costs for the care of children born to parents unable to provide for them.

In the heterogeneous society of the United States, reaching a national consensus about issues tied closely to sexual and religious mores is a major task. In recent years it has been made more difficult by a lack of political leadership and the lack of an official national framework in which to discuss and resolve the many ethical and emotional issues that surround human reproduction.

Every American pays the price for the absence of a national commitment to good reproductive health. Many of the unwanted births in this country have long-term deleterious effects on the lives of the women and girls who experience them as well as on their families and communities. The majority of unintended pregnancies occur in teenagers and young women who often have few financial resources and are uninsured for childbirth. They are less likely to receive adequate prenatal care and are at greater risk of giving birth prematurely. As a result, it is not unusual for their babies to need more intensive care. Hospitals annually incur $7 billion in debt for unreimbursed maternity care, and that debt is passed along to the public. Furthermore, studies have demonstrated that the unplanned-for child continues to need more support from public assistance programs, sometimes for many years.

There exists a dichotomy in reproductive health today. On one

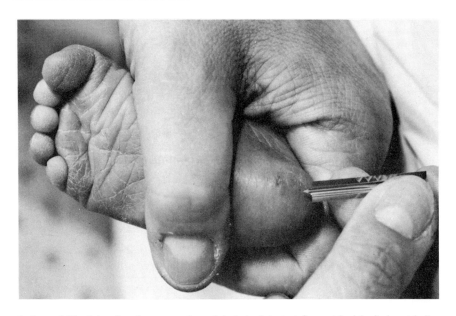

A drop of blood is taken from a newborn baby's heel to test for certain inherited metabolic diseases. Early treatment for some disorders results in a healthy child. Credit: National Institute of Child Health and Human Development

hand are the many pregnancies that are unplanned and economically and emotionally stressful; on the other is the substantial problem of infertility and the willingness of many infertile couples to pay thousands of dollars for help getting pregnant. Before the first test tube baby was born in 1978, the only available techniques to overcome infertility were artificial insemination, drugs to induce ovulation, and surgery to repair the reproductive tract in men and women. Since then, an entire "baby-making" industry that uses the latest in reproductive technologies has sprung into existence. It is an area in which costs are high and success rates are low, but because the industry is privately funded, it operates largely without public scrutiny.

Although concern about infertility is on the rise, the inability to settle the ethical and emotional issues related to human reproduction has severely slowed breakthroughs regarding the fertilization process and the early development of the human embryo. Generally, major research in the United States is funded by the federal government. But because research on fertility and the early stages of life might mean using excess embryos from in vitro fertilization programs, right-to-life groups protested against government support of such studies when they were originally proposed in the mid-1970s.

In 1978 some attempt was made to resolve the conflict by establishing an Ethical Advisory Board (which subsequently became known as the Ethics Advisory Board or EAB), but the EAB accomplished little before its funding and charter ended in 1980. Without a mechanism for resolving the ethical issues associated with reproductive research, federal funding became unavailable. The few studies that have been conducted have been funded by private organizations. The result has been an unofficial but effective moratorium on the development of new knowledge and no public oversight of private efforts, which include a variety of infertility interventions and the manipulation of eggs and embryos.

The United States is not alone in facing these new ethical and social concerns. Although most other developed countries have surpassed the United States in providing adequate family planning, improved contraception, and good prenatal care, our ethical questions and concerns arising from new reproductive technologies are the same. They include:

• When does human life begin?

• Up to what stage of embryo development should research be allowed?

• Who owns the cryopreserved embryos when the parents have divorced or died?

• Is research on early-stage embryos ethically acceptable?

• Is it permissible to create embryos or to use excess embryos specifically for research purposes?

Committees and commissions in every involved country have wrestled with these questions and at least 85 statements on the new reproductive technologies have been issued, but in this country many questions remain unresolved. Some concerns will fade with experience and the passage of time, but others will need thoughtful analysis and new public policies.

INFERTILITY

For every 12 married couples in this country who achieve a pregnancy when they choose to, there is a couple who cannot have a baby because of some childbearing impairment. According to the National Center for Health Statistics, in 1988 at least 2.3 million couples experienced infertility. Although the center's National Survey of Family

Growth revealed that infertility overall had declined somewhat since 1965, it also found that the problem had increased from 4 to 7 percent in young women in their early 20s, a rise attributed largely to the spread of sexually transmitted diseases in this highly sexually active age group.

Conception cannot occur if one of the essential reproductive components is lacking: ovulation; enough competent sperm at the site of fertilization; and at least one functioning fallopian tube, where the egg can be fertilized and then, as it develops, be transported to the hormone-primed uterus.

Physiological causes of infertility include the absence of ovulation; sperm that may be deficient in number or in ability to reach the egg; and damage to the fallopian tubes, uterus, or cervix. In women the inflammatory infections of sexually transmitted diseases (STDs) leave scar tissue that can affect the functioning of the fallopian tubes and uterus. In men such infections may impair sperm production and quality. Less common is infertility caused by an abnormal interaction between the sperm and the woman's cervical mucus.

In 90 percent of infertility cases the reason can be found through a series of tests, and approximately half the couples treated for infertility will become pregnant at least once, and most of them will successfully birth a child. Some causes, however, are more difficult to pinpoint. Sperm quality, for example, is hard to measure, and even when it appears to be the source of the infertility, too few treatments exist for overcoming sperm deficiencies. Similarly, not enough is known about the process of sperm movement through the female reproductive system or how sperm recognize, penetrate, and bond with the egg.

Efforts to circumvent unknown or intractable obstacles to reproduction have led to the development of new reproductive technologies: artificial insemination, treatments for stimulating ovulation, fallopian tube reconstruction, in vitro fertilization (IVF), and gamete intrafallopian transfer (GIFT). In IVF a number of eggs are fertilized by sperm outside the body and several of the healthy embryos that may result are returned to the uterus to continue their growth. In GIFT, sperm and two or three healthy eggs are injected together near the end of the fallopian tube, where fertilization would normally occur. The success rates for GIFT are somewhat higher than for IVF.

Clinics to treat infertility have existed for decades and have had considerable success treating ovulation disorders. With the advent of IVF in 1978 and the more recent development of GIFT in the mid-1980s, the desire of infertile couples to have children has led to the burgeoning of centers specializing in these two techniques. According to a recent survey by the Subcommittee on Regulation, Business Opportunities, and Energy of the U.S. House of Representatives' Committee on Small Business, by late 1988 there were 190 such centers in the United States. Forty opened in 1987 alone.

Each attempt at IVF or GIFT can cost $4,000 or more, with some women undergoing four to six attempts. Success rates are low. On average the 1987 and 1988 success rate for IVF births per stimulated cycle was 9 percent. For GIFT the success rate per stimulated cycle was 11 percent in 1987 and 16 percent in 1988. Some of the clinics so far have produced no births. The Office of Technology Assessment reports that only one in ten couples who undergo IVF or GIFT procedures takes home a baby.

IVF and GIFT have become far more popular than even their advocates expected. Women disrupt their lives for months, making trip after trip to the fertility center for hormone treatment, egg harvesting, and then implantation of developing embryos for a chance at having a biological child. Despite their efforts, a large proportion of them never take home a baby.

The increased number of fertility clinics offering IVF and GIFT may make these techniques somewhat more accessible, but their proliferation and the advent of commercial pressures have brought new concerns. Questions have been raised regarding the truthfulness of clinics' advertised success rates, the high costs, whether they will continue to limit the technique to those who can afford it, and what tests are in place to make certain that donated sperm is free from serious infections.

As new technologies become available that make it possible to choose an embryo's gender or to alter its genetic makeup, new ethical concerns are bound to arise. At the root of these issues is the fact that there are no controls regarding quality and safety because the technology has been developed with private funds. In the absence of a federal role in the development of reproductive technologies, the only controls are those of supply and demand.

CONTRACEPTION

In contrast to couples who cannot have the baby they want are the many more women who each month fear that they are pregnant. For the main part these women and girls are not using contraceptives because of their side effects or because they have not found a method that is reliable or easy enough to use. Despite current assumptions that anxiety about acquired immune deficiency syndrome (AIDS) has encouraged a decrease in intercourse among young unmarried Americans, a 1987 survey by Ortho Pharmaceutical Corporation uncovered little indication that levels of sexual activity have decreased since 1982. The survey also found that more than 3 million fertile, sexually active women in the United States do not use contraception at all. And of those who do, a considerable percentage use less effective nonmedical methods such as rhythm, withdrawal, or douching.

The proportion of women of childbearing age in the United States who use no contraception is much higher than it is in other developed countries. Rates of childbearing and abortion also are greater in the United States. A recent study by the Alan Guttmacher Institute examined the relationships between contraceptive use and public family planning policies and programs in the United States and in 19 other countries with similar economic, social, and demographic backgrounds. The study found that the United States leads the industrialized world in the number of abortions and unplanned births per capita.

According to the Guttmacher study, differences in contraceptive use among the 20 countries reflect differences in how contraceptive care is offered. Outside the United States contraceptive care generally is integrated into primary health services, making it less expensive and readily available at convenient and familiar locations. Family planning clinics offer counseling, extended hours, and a broad range of contraceptive methods to the general population. In the United States such clinics are set up chiefly to serve the poor and often are perceived as offering a lower standard of care.

In addition, other nations offer reliable contraceptive methods that are not available in the United States because of liability considerations and the abortion controversy. Contraceptives often are inexpensive or free in other countries. There is also substantially greater dissemination of information about contraception and sexuality through advertising, publicity, and education. Birth control is treated in a nonemotional way as a routine health matter.

Instead of the decrease in contraceptive costs and the increase in variety that observers had expected to see in the United States by 1990, prices are rising and access to some methods, such as IUDs, has sharply declined. In the early 1970s, 13 pharmaceutical firms were active world-wide in contraceptive research and development; by 1987 that number had dropped to four, with only two located in the United States.

U.S. interest in developing contraceptive methods has been flagging for some years. Insufficient funding, a fading concern about population growth, the regulatory hurdles of the Food and Drug Administration (FDA), less scientific interest, and the abortion controversy have all had a negative impact. Moreover, the prevalence of product litigation has dealt a severe blow to the pharmaceutical industry, which was already unenthusiastic about its contraceptive business.

But modest efforts to change the situation are under way. The Norplant implantable contraceptive is expected to be available by early 1991 in the United States, and FDA requirements for testing contraceptive steroids recently were made almost identical to the testing requirements for other drugs. Increased federal funding also has been proposed. A study published in February 1990 showed that taxpayers save $4.40 for every public dollar spent to provide birth control services to women who otherwise might not have access to them.

Although professionals are concerned, the decline in contraceptive availability has received little notice either from the U.S. public or from policymakers. The misconception that many methods are readily available appears to still exist, but the increased number of abortions is a noteworthy signal of poor contraceptive accessibility.

TEENAGE PARENTHOOD

More than 1 million adolescent girls in the United States become pregnant each year. For a pregnant teenager the considerable gap between her ability to reproduce and her ability to be self-sufficient causes a range of problems that will affect her life, her infant, and her community for years. More than 400,000 of these pregnant teenagers obtain abortions and approximately 470,000 of them give birth. Their rate of miscarriage is high. Most of the births are to unmarried teenagers, and nearly half of those new mothers are not yet 18. Despite an overall decline in the U.S. birth rate and despite the fact that teenage sexual activity in this country is similar to that of other westernized countries, the rate of adolescent pregnancy, childbearing, and abortion is still substantially higher in the United States. In this country girls under age 15 are at least five times more likely to have a baby than girls their age in other countries.

A 1987 study by the National Research Council Panel on Adolescent Pregnancy and Childbearing reported: "For teenage parents and their children, prospects for a healthy and independent life are significantly reduced. Young mothers, in the absence of adequate nutrition and appropriate prenatal care, are at a heightened risk of pregnancy complications and poor birth outcomes. . . . The infants of teenage mothers also face greater health and developmental risks."

The study also noted that adolescent parents are more likely to experience chronic unemployment and inadequate income and that they and their children are "highly likely to become dependent on public assistance and to remain dependent longer. . . ." It concluded that "in both human and monetary terms, it is less costly to prevent a pregnancy than to cope with its consequences." Consider this finding by the Alan Guttmacher Institute: In 1985 families started by a teenage birth absorbed approximately 53 percent of the total expenditures of the three major public programs for families—Aid to Families with Dependent Children (AFDC), food stamps, and Medicaid.

Aside from the personal and public costs of the epidemic of children having children, the unflagging rate of adolescent pregnancy in the United States is a case study for the argument for better contraception and better dissemination of information about sexual matters and contraception. It also illustrates what can happen when a nation does not deal directly with these issues. The social factors that contribute to an unintended early pregnancy have been identified, and a variety of policies, programs, and studies to alter some of these factors are under way. Until such interventions prove successful, however, the most reliable strategy for reducing the number of unintended pregnancies among sexually active teenagers is to encourage the use of contraception.

Not enough is known about how to make adolescents more precisely aware of the social and physical consequences of intercourse, including the dangers of sexually transmitted diseases. Sex education at home and at school appears to be easily overridden by the powerful sex-promotion messages of television and advertising. At least one survey indicates that Americans approve of condom advertising, but a national consensus about advertising to promote responsible attitudes toward sex has not been sought, largely out of fear of opposition from some religious groups.

PRENATAL CARE

Whether her pregnancy was planned or not, a woman or adolescent has a much better chance of having a healthy baby if she receives even a minimum of prenatal care. Such care appears to be especially important to both mother and child when the mother is at increased risk of medical or social problems. Prenatal care is also cost-effective because it significantly reduces the danger of having a low birthweight infant with its concomitant need for expensive medical treatment. Prenatal care also increases the baby's chance of surviving. In the poorest neighborhoods of New York City, for example, where many mothers receive little or no prenatal care, the mortality rate for newborns is more than twice that of the rest of the city.

Although the importance of prenatal care has been well established, during the 1980s its use in the United States declined. In 1985, 33 percent of all U.S. babies were born to mothers who did not obtain the recommended minimum amount of prenatal care, 25 percent were born to mothers who started care only after their third month of pregnancy, and 5 percent were born to women who began prenatal care in their last trimester or received no care at all. And 1985 was the sixth consecutive year in which no progress was made in reducing the number of women in the final group. Among blacks, those receiving little or no care increased from 8.8 percent in 1980 to 10.3 percent in 1985.

Despite the fact that the United States spends more per person for prenatal care than any other industrialized nation, barriers to such care obviously still exist, and the system is not working well. There is controversy about the content, costs, and effectiveness of the various public prenatal care programs. What constitutes good care has not been clearly defined, and the lack of a universal definition contributes to the dispute. Other questions have yet to be answered: Should care be measured by the number of visits or by what takes place during those visits? Should care entail only scheduled medical appointments, or should it include a range of educational and nutritional services in a setting that is flexible and appropriate to the cultural background of the community? Are the components of the care useful to the women being served? What are the best ways to draw women into care? What prevents women from seeking prenatal care?

ETHICAL ISSUES

Research on the earliest stages of life in animals and in humans has made it possible to fertilize human eggs in the laboratory and to store frozen embryos indefinitely. Recombinant DNA technology is providing tools for identifying genetic diseases in the embryo and for pinpointing the gene that determines the gender of a child. Studies of animal and human cells are allowing researchers to evaluate the chromosomal health of eggs and embryos in the hope of increasing the success of new reproductive techniques by choosing embryos that are normal.

Much of what we know about the reproductive process has been learned from research on animals, particularly farm animals. Technologies such as artificial insemination and the transfer, freezing, and division of embryos were originally developed for agricultural purposes. Newer technologies, such as determining the gender of embryos, growing embryos in the laboratory, and transferring genes, are being attempted with both animal and human cells. Two laboratories have altered the genetic composition of animal embryo cells so that the cells won't recognize such pathogens as the herpes virus. Although many animal technologies have been adapted successfully to human use, important questions about human reproduction remain that cannot be answered by animal research.

The future of IVF is tied to embryo research. The success of IVF and embryo transfer, in fact, could be improved if it were possible to determine whether the embryo was normal. The manipulation of embryos and studies of embryonic cells have led this and other countries into an area of ethics that is only sketchily charted. Some theologians, right-to-life groups, and others argue that life begins at the moment an egg is fertilized and that an embryo should have all the rights and protections accorded any other human being. Some say that an embryo has no human rights whatever. Others believe that research on embryos not used for implantation may be morally problematic but not without solution, much like using experimental treatments on terminally ill patients.

When federal regulations on fetal research were issued in 1975, their intent was to treat all fetuses equally after implantation, regardless of gestational age or whether abortion was intended. The commission that helped develop the regulations realized, however, that conflicts would inevitably develop between the obligation to treat all fetuses equally and the obligation to benefit individuals and society through fetal research. So the Ethics Advisory Board (EAB) was established within the U.S. Department of Health, Education, and Welfare to advise the department about the ethical acceptability of research proposals involving human subjects. The issue of embryo research was assigned to the EAB in 1978. A report favoring federal funding of research on the safety and efficacy of IVF as an infertility treatment was issued by the EAB in 1979.

Because medical researchers rely heavily on federal funding, the demise of the EAB in 1980 because its funding was not renewed and its charter was allowed to lapse was viewed by most U.S. scientists as a de facto ban on fetal research. As a result, very few new studies have since been proposed for federal funding. Some research is supported by private institutions, but the absence of the EAB has severely limited research on reproduction. It also has meant that ethically sensitive research is being performed without federal oversight and public input.

Without an EAB the federal government has had no way to evaluate the current ethical standards associated with reproductive technologies. Such an evaluation could examine the ethical implications of present and future public policies regarding artificial insemination, GIFT and IVF, egg donation, studies on embryo health, cryopreservation of both eggs and embryos, and other treatments for infertility or genetic diseases. It could then establish guides to research and clinical care in these areas.

To encourage more responsible conception, research and development on better contraceptives will have to be encouraged by policies that somehow protect both the consumer and the developer. In addition, long-term programs are needed to make the use of contraceptives less expensive and more of a social norm.

As Kenneth Ryan emphasized at the 1988 Institute of Medicine's annual meeting, these problems regarding reproductive health raise not only major scientific and clinical care issues but also vital public concerns that can best be addressed and resolved by the development of government policy.

REFERENCES

Fletcher, J.C., and K.J. Ryan. 1988. Federal regulations for fetal research: a case for reform. Law, Medicine & Health Care. 15:3.

Forrest, J.D., and R.R. Fordyce. 1988. U.S. women's contraceptive attitudes and practice: how have they changed in the 1980s? Family Planning Perspectives. 20(3)112-118.

Forrest, J.D., and S. Singh. 1990. Public-sector savings resulting from expenditures for contraceptive services. Family Planning Perspectives. 22(1):6-15.

Harkness, C. 1987. *The Infertility Book*. San Francisco: Volcano Press.

Institute of Medicine. 1988. *Prenatal Care: Reaching Mothers, Reaching Infants*. Sarah S. Brown, ed., Washington, D.C.: National Academy Press.

Jones, E.F., J.D. Forrest, S.K. Henshaw, et al. 1988. Unintended pregnancy, contraceptive practice and family planning services in developed countries. Family Planning Perspectives. 20(2):53-67.

Lincoln, R., and L. Kaeser. 1988. Whatever happened to the contraceptive revolution? Family Planning Perspectives. 20(1):20-24.

McShane, P.M. 1987. In vitro fertilization, GIFT and related technologies—hope in a test tube. In *Women & Health*. 13:31-46. Binghamton, N.Y.: The Haworth Press.

National Institutes of Health. 1989. Sex can cause more than AIDS. Healthline. August:3-4.

National Research Council. 1987. *Risking the Future: Adolescent Sexuality, Pregnancy, and Childbearing*. Washington, D.C.: National Academy Press.

Powledge, T.M. 1987. Reproductive technologies and the bottom line. In *Women & Health*. 13:203-209. Binghamton, N.Y.: The Haworth Press.

Raymond, C.A. 1988. In vitro fertilization enters stormy adolescence as experts debate the odds. Journal of the American Medical Association. 259(4):464.

Silverman, J., A. Torres, and J.D. Forrest. 1987. Barriers to contraceptive services. Family Planning Perspectives. 19(3):94-102.

Singh, S. 1986. Adolescent pregnancy in the United States: an interstate analysis. Family Planning Perspectives. 18(5):210-226.

United States Department of Health, Education, and Welfare, Ethics Advisory Board. 1979. *HEW Support of Research Involving Human In Vitro Fertilization and Embryo Transfer*. May 4.

Walters, L. 1987. Ethics and new reproductive technologies: an international review of committee statements. Hastings Center Report, Special Supplement. June.

Wallach, E.E. 1988. Testimony at the Hearing on Consumer Protection Issues Involving In Vitro Fertilization Clinics, before the House Subcommittee on Regulation and Business Opportunities. Washington, D.C. June 1.

Wyden, R. 1989. Opening remarks and testimony at the Hearing on Consumer Protection Issues Involving In Vitro Fertilization Clinics, before the House Subcommittee on Regulation, Business Opportunities, and Energy, Washington, D.C. March 9.

2

Infertility

On one hand, the United States has an extremely high rate of unwanted pregnancies; on the other, it has a large number of couples who want to have babies but are unable to conceive. Adoption is no longer a widely available solution, and for some couples it is not desirable because they want a biological tie with their child. About 50 percent of these couples are taking advantage of the increasing variety of new technologies to improve their chances of conceiving. A small but growing proportion are seeking help from the new reproductive techniques of in vitro fertilization (IVF) and gamete intrafallopian transfer (GIFT).

This chapter describes the process of human reproduction, the common and not-so-common causes of infertility, and the ways that reproductive disorders are diagnosed and treated. The issue of using frozen semen in artificial insemination by donor in order to protect the recipient and her offspring from sexually transmitted diseases and from AIDS is also outlined. The chapter focuses particularly on IVF and GIFT, how they are performed and for what reasons. The concentration is on these two treatments because clinics offering them are proliferating rapidly and without the accompanying development of quality control standards. Some clinics and physicians have been accused of confusing or misleading patients about their success rates and about which procedures are the most appropriate therapies. Existing avenues that could be utilized to establish standards for the performance of IVF and GIFT centers are noted.

HOW COMMON IS INFERTILITY?

Infertility is defined by physicians as not being able to conceive after 12 months of unprotected intercourse or being unable to carry a fetus to term. According to the 1988 National Survey of Family Growth by the National Center for Health Statistics, the number of infertile couples with no children (primary infertility) doubled since the National Fertility Survey in 1965, from 500,000 to 1 million. The increase was offset, however, by a drop in the number of couples who became infertile after having one or more children (secondary infertility). Using the survey as a basis, epidemiologists estimated the total number of all married couples in the United States experiencing infertility at 2.3 million, or 8 percent, which means about one married couple in 12 is infertile.

The escalation in primary infertility was most obvious among young women aged 20 to 24. In 1965, 4 percent in this age group were infertile; by 1988 that figure had risen to 7 percent. Many observers believe that the increase is due primarily to the prevalence of sexually transmitted diseases, such as gonorrhea and chlamydia, in this very sexually active segment of the population. Infertility among such young couples is significant because women at this age have one-third of the babies born in the United States.

THE PROCESS OF HUMAN REPRODUCTION

At birth the two ovaries of a baby girl will contain all the egg cells, or oocytes, needed for ovulation during her lifetime. A million oocytes may be present at birth, but the number will decline over time and only 300 to 500 actually will be ovulated. For an oocyte to develop into a mature egg and for ovulation to occur each month, a cycle of synchronized hormonal signals gets under way at puberty. Ovulation is the release of the egg from the ovary. The egg is captured by the tentaclelike overhanging fimbriae of the fallopian tube, or oviduct, which is connected to the uterus. Fertilization of the egg by the sperm takes place in the fallopian tube.

Over the next few days the egg is transported to the uterus, which has been primed to nurture the embryo if the egg is fertilized. If fertilization does not occur and no embryo is implanted in the uterine lining, a decline in hormone production will cause the blood-engorged lining to slough off. The superfluous tissue and blood are then expelled by uterine

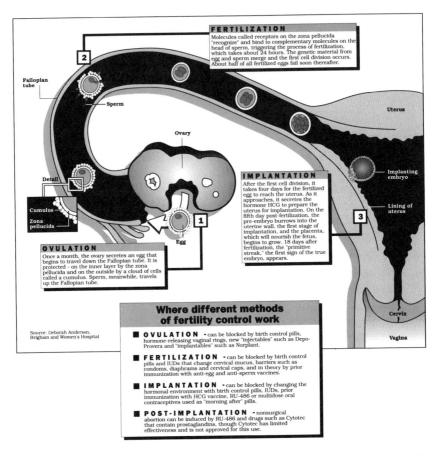

FERTILIZATION
Molecules called receptors on the zona pellucida "recognize" and bind to complementary molecules on the head of sperm, triggering the process of fertilization, which takes about 24 hours. The genetic material from egg and sperm merge and the first cell division occurs. About half of all fertilized eggs fail soon thereafter.

Fallopian tube

Sperm

Ovary

Uterus

Detail

Cumulus

Zona pellucida

Egg

IMPLANTATION
After the first cell division, it takes four days for the fertilized egg to reach the uterus. As it approaches, it secretes the hormone HCG to prepare the uterus for implantation. On the fifth day post-fertilization, the pre-embryo burrows into the uterine wall, the first stage of implantation, and the placenta, which will nourish the fetus, begins to grow. 18 days after fertilization, the "primitive streak," the first sign of the true embryo, appears.

Implanting embryo

Lining of uterus

OVULATION
Once a month, the ovary secretes an egg that begins to travel down the Fallopian tube. It is protected - on the inner layer by the zona pellucida and on the outside by a cloud of cells called a cumulus. Sperm, meanwhile, travels up the Fallopian tube.

Cervix

Vagina

Source: Deborah Anderson, Brigham and Women's Hospital

Where different methods of fertility control work

■ **OVULATION** - can be blocked by birth control pills, hormone-releasing vaginal rings, new "injectables" such as Depo-Provera and "implantables" such as Norplant.

■ **FERTILIZATION** - can be blocked by birth control pills and IUDs that change cervical mucus, barriers such as condoms, diaphrams and cervical caps, and in theory by prior immunization with anti-egg and anti-sperm vaccines.

■ **IMPLANTATION** - can be blocked by changing the hormonal environment with birth control pills, IUDs, prior immunization with HCG vaccine, RU-486 or multidose oral contraceptives used as "morning after" pills.

■ **POST-IMPLANTATION** - nonsurgical abortion can be induced by RU-486 and drugs such as Cytotec that contain prostaglandins, though Cytotec has limited effectiveness and is not approved for this use.

Credit: The Boston Globe/Neil C. Pinchin

contractions, which results in menstrual bleeding. This cycle is repeated every month unless the egg is fertilized and implants in the uterus.

In the male the continuous secretion of hormones is responsible for the constant production of spermatozoa in the testes from puberty through adulthood. For a sperm to grow from its earliest stage to maturity requires approximately 72 days. Usually, each ejaculation contains tens of millions of sperm.

On the surface the fertilization of an egg by a sperm seems simplicity itself. Propelled by the whipping motion of their tails, sperm swim through the mucus of the vagina and cervix, into the uterus of the female, and up into the fallopian tubes where, if ovulation has just occurred, they will encounter an egg ready for fertilization. For an egg to be fertilized successfully, it must be penetrated by a single sperm within 24 to 68 hours after ovulation. Although each ejaculation usually contains millions of spermatozoa, only a few hundred enter the uterus and make their way into the fallopian tubes.

Human eggs, like those of other mammals, are covered with a thick translucent layer called the zona pellucida, which the sperm must penetrate to reach the egg. Once viewed simply as an impediment to fertilization, the zona pellucida, research has revealed, functions as a sophisticated biological security system that chemically controls the entry of sperm into the egg and protects the fertilized egg from additional sperm.

Each healthy egg and sperm carries a single set of chromosomes— some three feet of DNA—drawn from the genetic endowment of the person producing it. At fertilization the maternal and paternal sets of chromosomes join to form a full complement of DNA and the egg becomes a zygote. If a second sperm were able to fertilize the egg, the extra set of chromosomes would produce an abnormal zygote that would not survive.

As the zygote moves slowly down the long, slender fallopian tube, it divides into two identical cells called blastomeres, each containing a complete set of genes. If the blastomeres are separated, they develop into identical twins, although that is not the only way identical twins can form. This ability to develop into two complete individuals has become an important factor in the reproductive technologies used in modern animal husbandry, in which blastomeres are divided to produce two offspring instead of one. Usually the blastomeres simply multiply and the resulting four cells divide in turn. Three to four days after fertilization, while this cluster of cells is still in the oviduct en route to the uterus, it can be described correctly as a blastocyst, conceptus, preembryo, or preimplantation embryo. For simplicity most physicians and clinic staff refer to the fertilized egg as an embryo, regardless of its stage of development.

On about the fourth or fifth day, the cluster reaches the uterus and breaks out of the zona pellucida; by day six or seven, it begins to embed itself in the uterine wall. When the embryo reaches the four- to eight-cell stage, the genes in its cells start the process of differentiation that eventually results in complex organs and tissues. It is only on about the eighteenth day after fertilization that the "primitive streak," the first evidence of a spinal cord, emerges and the cluster of cells can be called a true embryo. If a duplicate primitive streak develops, the result is twins; if the streaks are joined, Siamese twins occur. After the first differentiation of the major organ systems is completed, the embryo may be properly termed a fetus.

WHEN THE SYSTEM DOESN'T WORK

Simple as this process may appear, as any infertile couple knows, there are many points at which it can fail. The average chance of impregnation occurring in any given menstrual cycle is about 20 to 30 percent and that decreases as the woman grows older. To succeed, all the components of fertility must be in place: The woman must have at least one ovary and ovulation must occur; at least one fallopian tube must be capable of drawing in the egg and moving it to the uterus; enough competent sperm must reach the fertilization site within 24 hours of ovulation; and the uterus must be properly primed by hormones to accept and nourish the embryo. The entire process is orchestrated according to cycles of interaction between the hypothalamus and pituitary gland in the brain and the ovaries.

SEEKING THE CAUSE

When a couple has been unable to conceive after months of trying, they usually look to their family physician or the woman's gynecologist for help, since women visit their gynecologists more often than their male partners visit their physicians. According to a 1988 report on infertility by the congressional Office of Technology Assessment (OTA), as much as 80 percent of the basic treatments for infertility are given by the woman's gynecologist. The male partner usually is referred to a urologist for an infertility evaluation. If the problem persists, however, an increasing number of couples look to clinics or group practices that specialize in treating infertility. Because the disorder can have a variety of complex causes and can affect either partner, a team of specialists is generally considered to provide more skilled resources for thorough evaluation and treatment.

The best sources for such infertility treatment programs are medical schools, large group practices or health maintenance organizations, and large hospitals.

In addition to a medical and sexual history and a physical examination, infertility clinics use a battery of testing procedures to diagnose the cause of infertility. The most common are semen analysis; a test of sperm penetration ability; records of basal body temperatures for several months; cervical mucous examination; hormone monitoring; endometrial biopsy; X-ray studies of the female reproductive tract; direct visualization of the uterus and cervix by hysteroscope; direct visualization of the uterus, fallopian tubes, and ovaries through a laparoscope; and a study of the interaction of semen with the cervical mucus.

DAMAGE TO THE REPRODUCTIVE TRACT

Increasingly common as causes of infertility are blockages and adhesions that interfere with the normal role of the ovaries and fallopian tubes. Even minor adhesions can prevent the delicate functioning of the reproductive tract and are difficult, often impossible, to repair. These abnormalities may be the result of infection from a pelvic inflammatory disease (PID). The microbes that cause such an infection are passed from person to person via genital, oral, or anal contact. Genital infections may impair the fertility of men as well as women, but the extent to which men are affected is not known.

One factor that can increase the risk of PID is the use of an intrauterine device, or IUD. These effective contraceptives should be used only by women in mutually monogamous relationships who do not have a medical history of sexually transmitted infections.

The OTA estimates that 20 percent of all infertility is due to sexually transmitted diseases (STDs). The National Institute of Allergy and Infectious Diseases says that chlamydia and gonorrhea caused infertility in nearly 500,000 women in 1988, or about 40 percent of the 2.3 million infertile couples in the United States. These two diseases are responsible for more than two-thirds of the cases of inflammation-causing STDs treated every year. In fact, after the common cold and influenza, STDs are the most widespread infectious diseases in the United States. Chlamydia is the prevailing STD; the Centers for Disease Control (CDC) estimates that 4 million people had this infection during 1988.

Chlamydia is more difficult to detect than gonorrhea because its symptoms are not very noticeable. Like gonorrhea, if it is untreated or treated late, the inflammation it causes can scar delicate tissues and obstruct or deform the fine passages of the reproductive tract in men and women. Although both sexes can have chlamydia, it seems to affect female fertility more often.

Because many STDs do not always produce symptoms, they may be unknowingly transmitted to other sexual contacts. If both partners are not treated, they can reinfect one another. Unfortunately, each bout of infection substantially increases the likelihood of infertility.

OVULATION DISORDERS

Ovulation problems are a common cause of infertility, with the most obvious sign being a very irregular or nonexistent menstrual cycle. Detecting whether ovulation is taking place can be done several ways: charting the rise in basal body temperature that occurs just after ovulation, detecting the preovulatory surge of luteinizing hormone in the urine, or visualizing a large maturing egg in the ovary with ultrasound. These tests also help determine the source of the problem: hypothalamus, pituitary, or ovaries.

ENDOMETRIOSIS

The ability to conceive can be negatively affected by endometriosis, a disorder in which cells that ordinarily line the uterus grow in other areas of the body, such as in the ovaries, fallopian tubes, or the membranes that line the pelvis. One theory supposes that some blood and endometrial cells occasionally back up through the fallopian tubes and escape into the abdomen, from where they spread. Endometrial tissue has even been found in the lungs and lymph nodes. Not all women with endometriosis have symptoms. When the disease is symptomatic, however, it can produce painful menstruation, painful ovulation and intercourse, and infertility. Endometriosis can cause a wide range of effects, including interference with ovarian and fallopian tube functioning and changes in hormone levels. The likelihood of developing endometriosis increases with age.

CAUSES OF MALE INFERTILITY

Deficiencies in the number of sperm being produced and in their ability to move with vigor are observed in the male partners of 30 to 40 percent of infertile couples. Research on male infertility has progressed rapidly over the last decade, but more needs to be known about the reproductive physiology of the male and about diagnosing and treating sperm deficiencies. More research is also needed on the basic process of sperm movement through the female reproductive tract, although studies are beginning to provide important information on the biochemical interaction between sperm and the zona pellucida.

MEDICAL THERAPIES FOR WOMEN AND MEN

Medical treatments for female and male infertility can range from advice from a physician or nurse on how to pinpoint the time of ovulation to sophisticated drug regimens. A number of compounds are available to treat ovulatory dysfunctions and to improve semen quality in men who are infertile or subfertile. Infertile couples treated for ovulation disorders achieve pregnancy 50 to 60 percent of the time.

In women the compound used depends on the source of the disorder. Clomiphene citrate increases gonadotropin secretion, which stimulates the ovary. If the pituitary or the hypothalamus appears not to be functioning, the human menopausal gonadotropin or follicle-stimulating hormone is given to stimulate the ovary directly. If a high level of prolactin, the hormone responsible for milk production, is interfering with regular ovulation, bromocriptine is used to reduce the pituitary's prolactin secretion. If a faulty adrenal gland seems to be the cause, synthetic glucocorticoid hormones can restore ovulation. Some fertility specialists believe that taking progesterone may be necessary if that hormone is not produced adequately after ovulation.

In the substantial percentage of nonovulating women whose pituitary and ovaries are functioning but whose hypothalamus is releasing gonadotropin-releasing hormone (GnRH) at an abnormal frequency, or is not producing it at all, administering the missing hormone usually restores ovulation. This treatment and the research behind it are described in greater detail in Chapter 6.

Drug therapies such as continuous oral contraceptives or GnRH agonists are also being used to treat endometriosis, although their success may be variable. Currently popular is treatment with the drug danazol, a synthetic steroid that temporarily halts ovulation and menstruation by suppressing the normal secretion of the gonadotropins. Ovulation is stopped for four to six months either to temporarily arrest the endometriosis or to force it to regress, particularly from those areas where it is inhibiting reproduction. An examination via laparascope can then help determine the extent of endometrial regression.

In some cases the cause of infertility may be an immune or hostile reaction by the cervical mucus to the sperm; such a reaction can cause antibodies in the mucus to prevent proper sperm movement, decrease sperm viability, or adversely affect fertilization. Attempts to reduce the antibody levels in hostile cervical mucus have had only limited success; intrauterine insemination to bypass the cervical area is currently the preferred treatment method.

If the number of spermatozoa in semen is less than 20 million per milliliter, the likelihood of natural fertilization is reduced. Although the quality of the sperm, not the number, is most important, fertilization becomes statistically less likely as the number drops below 20 million. The causes of lowered sperm production can include hormone dysfunction, drug use, or damage to the reproductive tract. Hormone therapy may help. It is most effective when the cause of infertility is insufficient gonadotropin secretion. For some men a combination of human menopausal gonadotropin and human chorionic gonadotropin results in more normal sperm development. Hormone drugs such as clomiphene citrate and tamoxifen citrate can enhance the body's own production of the gonadotropins, which in turn act on the testes to generate sperm. If the hypothalamus is not secreting the rhythmic pulses of GnRH necessary to trigger sperm development, the treatment is a continuous administration of pulses of GnRH via a portable infusion pump.

SURGICAL TREATMENT FOR VARICOCELE

Varicoceles affect sperm count, motility, and structure in approximately 25 percent of infertile men. The condition forms when the valves of the vein fail to close behind the retreating flow of blood, causing blood to back up and pool and the vein to dilate. It occurs most often in the left testis, where the anatomical arrangement of the renal vein is thought to heighten the likelihood of dysfunction.

A varicocele probably affects fertility because the pool of blood raises the temperature in the scrotum. Sperm development is temperature sensitive and even a slight increase could have an adverse effect.

Whatever the actual mechanism, eliminating the backflow of blood into the testis can increase both the quality and the quantity of the ejaculate. The most common treatment of varicocele is a fairly simple operation in which the dysfunctional vein is tied off. A newer method uses an X-ray-guided catheter to place a balloon or coil in the distended vein in order to block the flow of blood. The true effectiveness of these treatments has not yet been established. In the months after treatment, semen quality does improve in about 75 percent of cases, but the improvement does not always result in a pregnancy. The percentage of men whose spouses become pregnant is smaller than the percentage whose sperm quality improves.

SURGICAL TREATMENT FOR WOMEN

Surgical treatment is available to cut or remove adhesions that have formed in the ovaries or fallopian tubes after an inflammation or injury from other causes, such as prior surgery. It is also an option for endometriosis that is severe or does not respond to drug therapy. Repairing deformities in such delicate structures, however, is difficult, and success rates are not high. Repairs in the fallopian tubes, for instance, are associated with an increased risk that if a pregnancy does occur it will be tubal or ectopic. The advent of microsurgery—operating under the magnification of a microscope—and the laser has helped to improve the chances of restoring these organs to normal functioning. The likelihood of success also greatly depends on the surgeon's skill and experience.

ARTIFICIAL INSEMINATION

One of the oldest and simplest treatments for infertility, artificial insemination is also one of the most successful. The OTA found in 1987 that 172,000 women underwent at least one cycle of artificial insemination from 1986 to 1987. The survey data suggest that live births were achieved in about one-third of the women who received this form of infertility therapy. The technique is designed to overcome problems such as insufficient number of sperm, sperm that are not active, or antibodies in the cervical mucus that make it hostile to sperm.

To prepare sperm for insemination, the semen sample is centrifuged, or "washed," to separate the sperm from other material in the semen. Some infertility clinics select the most active by using the "swim-up" technique. The washed sperm are placed under layers of a thick protein solution; the most vigorous sperm reach the top layer and are collected for use. The sperm concentrate is also treated with antibiotics to eliminate bacterial infections.

Because an egg is most susceptible to fertilization for approximately 24 hours after ovulation, insemination is planned to coincide with ovulation. A sperm sample is produced by the male partner, prepared, drawn into a syringe, and injected into the cervical canal leading to the uterus or into the uterus itself. Although methods may vary, clinics generally favor performing several inseminations during each fertile period to enhance the chance of success.

If the cause of infertility is the male partner's inability to produce sperm in the large numbers needed for fertilization and his condition does not respond to treatment, donor sperm are used.

In the past, fresh donor sperm were used by most infertility clinics. But in recent years medical scientists have recognized that semen can carry a variety of STDs, including AIDS. In response, the CDC, the Food and Drug Administration, and concerned professional organizations, such as the American Association of Tissue Banks, have formulated guidelines for screening donors and semen.

In the February 5, 1988, issue of the *Morbidity and Mortality Weekly Report*, the CDC strongly recommends that donated semen be frozen and quarantined for at least six months before use. Before the semen is used for artificial insemination, a blood sample taken at the time the semen was collected and a second blood sample taken a minimum of six months later should be tested for HIV antibody. Care must be taken to assure that both blood samples are from the same donor, the CDC advised, and donor semen should not be used unless both tests are negative. The CDC urged this approach to make it possible to detect infections that were incubating and not identifiable at the time of donation.

This federal action came almost two years after an article strongly recommending donor and semen screening appeared in the May 1986 *New England Journal of Medicine*. CDC infectious disease specialists Laurene Mascola and Mary E. Guinan demonstrated that there was substantial scientific evidence that STDs could be passed along through artificial insemination. They urged that a sexual history be taken from all semen donors, that donors be tested for syphilis and hepatitis B, and that the semen sample itself be examined for pathogenic organisms. They emphasized that donated semen should not be used until all tests were shown to be negative. Drs. Mascola and Guinan warned that the use of fresh semen "is clearly hazardous and should be discouraged, especially because of the risk of AIDS."

Although observers believe that most reputable fertility clinics and private physicians using artificial insemination are following the CDC guidelines, a number of practitioners may be still be using fresh sperm. Some believe that fresh semen achieves a higher pregnancy rate. Because fresh sperm remains viable for only a few hours, however, its use does not permit thorough testing for disease organisms. Instead, the physician must rely on a personal evaluation of the donor. Most donors are single and under age 35, the age group with the highest reported incidence of STDs, a fact that underscores the importance of using only frozen sperm from carefully screened donors.

NEW FERTILIZATION PROCEDURES

In Vitro Fertilization

In 1978 a normal baby was born in England after fertilization in a test tube. The feat marked the culmination of two decades of research on reproduction as well as the availability of several new medical technologies. Although the technique has since been refined, the approach used by gynecologist Patrick Steptoe, of the Oldham and District Hospital in Lancashire, and reproductive physiologist Robert G. Edwards, of Cambridge University, has remained essentially the same. Today in vitro fertilization (IVF) is used chiefly when infertility is caused by tubal damage in the woman, male infertility, endometriosis, problems with cervical mucous quality, or the presence of antisperm antibodies or when infertility cannot be explained. IVF is designed to bypass such obstacles because fertilization is conducted in a laboratory dish, where its completion or failure can be observed.

In IVF, hormone drugs are used to induce the ovulation of more than one egg, the eggs are removed from developed ovarian follicles, prepared sperm are added to those harvested oocytes, and, if fertilization is successful, the growing embryo is placed into the uterus. Simple in concept, IVF depends a great deal on other new technologies for its success: radioimmunoassay to monitor ovulation via hormone levels, ultrasound to visualize egg development, and laparoscopy to retrieve the eggs with a needle aspirator through a tiny incision in the abdomen. Eggs can also be collected nonsurgically via the vagina, with the aspirator guided by ultrasound, an approach that has become widely used.

Because infertile patients may have a number of physiological disorders that reduce the chance of IVF success, several embryo transfers usually are necessary and several embryos are used in each implantation attempt. For this reason and to reduce the number of retrieval procedures, it has become common practice to use hormone drugs to induce the ovaries to produce as many oocytes as possible.

Not all the oocytes retrieved from the ovaries are suitable for fertilization. They may be immature or chromosomally abnormal (the latter condition also occurs when ovulation is spontaneous). Extra eggs are usually fertilized and the resulting embryos frozen and stored in case the first attempt at achieving a pregnancy fails.

Although cattle embryos have been frozen and used afterward with a high rate of success, freezing human embryos has not been as successful. The reasons are not clear because our knowledge of the human embryo is incomplete. Research on human embryos is not supported by government funding in the United States. As a result, medical scientists have had to draw largely on animal embryo research for information on some aspects of human reproduction. There are many important differences in the details of reproduction among mammals, and technology developed for other animals is not always transferable to humans.

After the eggs have been harvested, the male partner provides a sperm sample, which is prepared as it would be for artificial insemination. The most active sperm are chosen, counted to make sure enough are present for fertilization, and added to the eggs in a culture medium, which is then placed in an incubator. If the sperm are sufficiently vigorous and the egg is healthy and at the correct stage of maturity, fertilization and division occur within 48 hours. Eggs that have been successfully fertilized and are dividing are placed within the uterus of the female partner. Currently, fertility specialists use embryos at the four-cell stage of development. Dr. Edwards, who directs the Bourn Hall clinic in England, notes that no one yet has done a comparative study to determine the best stage at which to place human embryos in the uterus.

Experience has shown that the chance of a pregnancy occurring increases with the number of embryos placed in the uterus, and many IVF practitioners will use two or three, and sometimes as many as six or seven, embryos to achieve a single pregnancy. The likelihood of naturally occurring multiple births is slightly more than 1 percent; in IVF, multiple births occur considerably more frequently, at a rate 15 to 20 percent.

Gamete Intrafallopian Transfer

If at least one fallopian tube in an infertile woman is functioning, a variation of the IVF technique can be used. Gamete intrafallopian transfer (GIFT) is similar to IVF in its methods of ovarian stimulation, oocyte collection, and sperm preparation. But instead of fertilization taking place in a laboratory dish, three or four eggs and a large number of sperm are deposited via catheter into the ampulla section of the fallopian tube, the area where fertilization normally occurs. GIFT was developed on the theory that fertilization in the tubal environment was more natural and therefore more likely to occur than in a culture dish in a laboratory incubator.

A survey of the nation's IVF clinics and procedures by the congressional Subcommittee on Regulation, Business Opportunities, and Energy found that in 1988 the rate of live births per stimulated ovarian cycle was measurably higher for GIFT than for IVF. The overall success rate for IVF was 9 percent per stimulated cycle; for GIFT it was 16 percent.

GIFT has some drawbacks: Placing the eggs and sperm into the fallopian tubes is usually done via laparoscopy, which requires general anesthesia. Also, if a pregnancy does not occur, there is no way to know whether fertilization actually took place, which makes it difficult to establish a reason for the failure.

Setting Standards for the New Technologies

IVF and GIFT have evolved rapidly from being experimental techniques to becoming widely accepted clinical treatments. The methods have become more sophisticated, and the centers applying them have proliferated. From 1983 to 1987 the number of centers offering IVF grew from 10 to 167. Forty new clinics opened in 1987 alone. According to OTA estimates, in 1987 infertility was a $1 billion a year business; 7 percent of that, or $70 million, was spent on IVF. Each attempt to conceive through IVF and related methods costs from $4,000 to $7,000; the majority of infertile couples try at least one or two fertilization/implantation cycles. If the number of infertile young women continues to grow, it will further fuel the expansion of IVF/GIFT services.

Several months before the Subcommittee on Regulation, Business Opportunities, and Energy surveyed the IVF clinics in the United States, it held a hearing on consumer protection issues involving IVF clinics. At that June 1988 hearing, fertility specialist Richard P. Marrs told the committee and its chairman, Representative Ron Wyden of Oregon, that the dramatic growth of facilities offering new infertility therapies has intensified the need for licensing, for setting standards of optimal care, and for developing the regulatory measures necessary to protect patients and to improve the quality of the therapies. Because these technologies have advanced so swiftly and have been developed largely with private funds, neither their research nor their clinical application has been regulated by federal guidelines for research on human subjects.

States have the right to regulate important aspects of the new reproductive technologies and have done so in the case of artificial insemination by donor. While sperm-penetration tests must be performed by licensed physicians in licensed facilities, only a few states have specific statutes or licensing requirements for IVF and none has regulated the use of GIFT. Although almost all states require that clinical laboratories be certified, Dr. Marrs told the subcommittee that laboratories performing sperm separation, sperm preparation, embryo fertilization and incubation, and embryo freezing are not required to be licensed.

In the absence of federal and state controls, professional societies with members in the field of infertility care are formulating standards for IVF and GIFT. The first U.S. test tube baby was born in December 1981; in January 1984 the American Fertility Society published a one-page description of qualifications for the personnel, facilities, and ancillary support involved with in vitro fertilization. In July 1988 the society published standards for GIFT.

The American Association of Tissue Banks and the American College of Obstetricians and Gynecologists also have promulgated guidelines for the new infertility therapies. But no society or group has site inspection powers, and compliance with guidelines is entirely voluntary.

Insurance companies can influence therapy quality by setting standards for the treatments they cover, but insurers have been reluctant to include IVF in health plans because of the procedure's low success rates, potential high cost, and other variables. As of January 1989, five states had mandated such insurance coverage and another five were considering it. As more health insurance plans are being written to cover infertility treatments, insurers are expected to formulate a broad variety of requirements in an effort to assure adequate care. Any movement to provide insurance coverage for IVF and GIFT is expected to be slow, however, because such coverage is expected to add a considerable dollar amount to already increasing health plan costs.

PROTECTING THE CONSUMER

Concerned professionals have pinpointed three areas in the field of infertility treatment in which better quality control is needed to protect patients: the credentialing of personnel, the protocols for applying the new techniques, and the claims regarding success rates.

Physician Credentials

At present there is no credentialing process for physicians performing IVF and GIFT. In a November 1987 editorial in *Fertility and Sterility*, Dr. Richard E. Blackwell and 10 other obstetricians and gynecologists warned that few of the four-year residency programs in obstetrics and gynecology teach the skills needed for advanced infertility therapy, including those needed for IVF and GIFT. They pointed out that postgraduate courses without supervised, hands-on experience are not adequate preparation for applying new therapies. As they said:

> The lack of standards and absence of a credentialing process with IVF are equally disturbing. It has become commonplace for practitioners to visit academic or private IVF programs and then return to their hospitals and attempt to open IVF or GIFT programs. The motive for establishing such programs may not be a strong interest in IVF or the desire to fill a void in the community, but an attempt to increase its market share. Considering that half of the IVF programs that have been established in the country have no pregnancies, it would seem that the standards of practice are quite variable.

Using Procedures Appropriately

The physicians also noted that it is possible for couples and individuals seeking a solution to their infertility to receive evaluations that are too extensive or that are not complete. They recommended that such evaluations should be done one step at a time, with the less invasive (and least expensive) performed first and the invasive and more specialized procedures resorted to after conservative treatment has not succeeded. Moreover, they said that enough time should be allowed after each therapy for a pregnancy to occur.

In its report on infertility, the OTA made a similar assessment. Couples may be offered, as routine, treatments that are still experimental, the OTA said. Patients also may be offered procedures that have not been proved effective or safe or that are inappropriate for overcoming their particular infertility problem.

On one hand, some physicians or clinics are encouraging patients to undergo IVF or GIFT before less invasive treatments have been attempted; on the other, many centers are still not using the most advanced forms of infertility techniques, including the use of frozen donor sperm. The OTA estimates that the time lag for the dissemination of new technology may be as long as two years.

Defining IVF and GIFT Success

Of major concern to the public and professionals both inside and outside the fertility field is exactly how "success" is defined by IVF and GIFT centers. Some clinics have never produced a baby. Patients appearing before Representative Wyden's subcommittee described their experiences with clinics that claimed as their own success rates based on the experience of other centers.

Other witnesses at the hearing characterized clinics as not always explaining to prospective clients that the underlying infertility disorder and the age of the individual woman may have a significant effect on the outcome of the treatment, regardless of how successful IVF has been for some couples. Clinics with higher than average rates of success might be treating only patients under age 35 or patients with infertility disorders that are relatively easy to overcome. Moreover, couples eager to become parents may be allowed to assume that "success" means taking home a baby, when instead the clinic staff is referring to the establishment of a pregnancy.

The testimony led the subcommittee to launch its survey of this country's IVF clinics, their procedures, and their results. With a questionnaire developed with the help of the American Fertility Society, 224 clinics were polled in late 1988 by the subcommittee staff. Of the 190 centers that responded, 165 reported that they performed IVF and 146 provided complete data from 1987 and 1988.

From the data the subcommittee learned that the success rate of live births per stimulated ovulatory cycles was 9 percent for IVF in both 1987 and 1988. The success rate for GIFT was 11 percent in 1987 and 16 percent in 1988, based on the number of births per stimulated cycles. The data also showed that the number of patients seeking IVF and GIFT had increased from 10,598 patients in 1987 to 13,597 patients in 1988. In reporting on the success rates for this technology at a second hearing in March 1989, Representative Wyden cautioned:

> Success rates should not be viewed in a vacuum. Just as they can be abused to give patients false hopes of success, they can be misused to give them a falsely dismal view of IVF's successes. For example, clinics that treat the more difficult cases such as male infertility and older women can reflect lower success rates. But they may be the very clinics some patients need to treat their specific problems.

When IVF centers are new and do not have a track record to attract patients, they have been known to quote as their own the success rates for IVF and GIFT that are reported in the professional literature. The Wyden

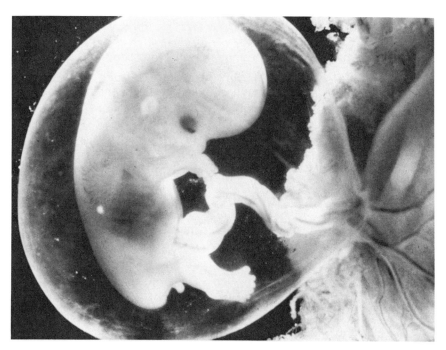

A photograph of a 12- to 14-week-old fetus inside the uterus demonstrates an important technique available to medical science for evaluating the reproductive process. Credit: National Institute of Child Health and Human Development

subcommittee discovered that a newly formed branch of an internationally known IVF center was advertising as its own successes the many births achieved by its parent organization. Representative Wyden observed:

> The subcommittee's investigation turned up instances of questionable advertising practices. Success rates are exaggerated, and consumers may be grossly misled. . . . At present, there is virtually no professional or government oversight of this booming industry. Any practitioner can hold himself out as a fertility specialist.

In the professional fertility literature, "clinical pregnancy" or "successful pregnancy" are the terms used when a positive fetal heartbeat is detected by ultrasound to confirm that an embryo has implanted and that a pregnancy has begun. Until recently, fertility specialists often preferred to use pregnancy data because they felt such data were the most accurate measure of success for the technique, but as Dr. Marrs noted in his testimony, there was no single format for reporting pregnancy outcome. For an infertile couple, the most meaningful figure is a clinic's "take-home baby rate."

Success after implantation depends almost entirely on the health of the embryo and, to a lesser degree, on the woman's physiological ability to carry a fetus to term. An abnormal egg or sperm, a faulty union between them, or a chance genetic mutation during the first stages of embryo development are common causes of unsuccessful implantation or spontaneous abortion, in nature or after IVF. A substantial percentage of embryo transfers do not become clinical pregnancies, and a substantial number of pregnancies do not result in a live birth. Many women will experience spontaneous abortions and some will develop ectopic pregnancies, which have to be terminated. Between October 1980 and July 1985, Dr. Edwards's IVF clinic achieved 767 clinical pregnancies, of which 500 were carried to term.

To confuse the layperson further, clinical pregnancy rates have been reported differently by different clinics: in terms of pregnancies per attempt to retrieve oocytes, pregnancies per fertilization, or pregnancies per transfer of embryo. The Wyden subcommittee chose to report the findings of its survey in terms of the number of live births that resulted from stimulated ovulatory cycles. The subcommittee staff selected this approach because stimulating the ovaries to produce eggs is the first step in the IVF process; they felt this was the fairest, most accurate basis on which to determine a success rate. In his testimony before the 1989 Wyden subcommittee hearing, Dr. Gary B. Ellis, then project director of the OTA infertility study, said the OTA agreed that the stimulated cycle was the soundest starting point from which to measure success rates.

The age of the woman is a factor in the success of IVF, with women over age 40 having fewer live births. Data based on the results of more than 8,000 embryo transfers in 1987 showed a 4 percent drop in the clinical pregnancy rate and a 5 percent increase in spontaneous abortion rates for women 40 and older. Although both percentages are small, together they indicate a lower IVF birth rate for women over 40.

In their editorial in *Fertility and Sterility*, Dr. Blackwell and his colleagues cautioned fertility professionals that it is misleading to claim a high pregnancy rate based on a small number of patients and on pregnancies determined by a blood test. It also is deceptive, they said, for a clinic to quote a high pregnancy rate based solely on its experience with young patients who have only tubal disease or to use as its overall success rate the pregnancies that occurred in a period when results were unusually good.

In late 1989 U.S. IVF clinics voted to make public the success rates of individual clinics based on uniform criteria. By making these rates available, the industry hoped to avoid the patient exploitation decried by its critics. Although the American Fertility Society had collected this information, it was not divulged, and some clinics were claiming success rates of 40 to 50 percent. After the Wyden subcommittee survey revealed that success rates were actually much lower, the industry agreed to publish its clinic-by-clinic figures. IVF clinic spokespersons cautioned, however, that an individual clinic's overall success rate is affected by the types of infertility it treats and the age of its patients. Clinics that treat the more difficult cases are likely to have a lower overall rate, despite the fact that on a matched-patient basis their rate of success might be as good or better than those clinics that turn away difficult cases.

Questions to Ask an IVF Clinic

Because of the difficulty of discovering the success record of a particular IVF center, the OTA suggests that before beginning IVF treatment patients might want to ask clinic personnel a number of questions, including:

• What is the center's live-birth rate per cycle of drug-stimulated ovulation? What is the clinic's success rate for patients of similar ages who have had similar types of infertility?

• Does the clinic implant all fertilized eggs or only those that appear capable of normal development? Does it limit the number of implanted fertilized eggs to minimize the risks associated with multiple births? Can the clinic freeze extra embryos for later attempts? What has been the clinic's rate of loss for those embryos?

• Does the clinic have an andrology referral source so the male partner can be correctly and fully evaluated?

• Does the clinic offer psychological counseling, or does it have a regular means of referral for those patients who seek such help? Is the counseling coordinated with the medical workup and transfer attempts to anticipate difficulties and disappointments?

• Is the program community based or is it a referral center? Referral centers are beginning to train local physicians to handle preliminary workups and ovulation inductions, so patients need travel to the main center fewer times.

• Does the clinic offer assistance in obtaining the highest possible insurance reimbursement for its patients? What has been the reimbursement experience of other patients with similar insurance plans? Does the clinic offer a sliding-fee scale for patients with low incomes?

Some Approaches for Protecting Consumers

A traditional means of establishing and encouraging the use of standards for high-quality medical care is the use of consensus conferences. As the OTA noted in its report, conferences have been sponsored by professional societies, government agencies, and insurance companies in an effort to develop protocols for medical care in order to safeguard research subjects and patients. A logical goal for such a meeting, the OTA suggested, would be the development of a protocol to determine which infertility treatment is the best approach for a given patient. To protect consumers further, critics say, there is a need to establish the difference between experimental and therapeutic treatments and to upgrade the current minimum practice standards set by professional societies.

Much of the power to protect the public health lies with the states. Avenues open to them include the licensing of health care personnel and facilities, certificate-of-need laws, statutes and regulations that relate to medical practice, and controls regarding professional liability. The OTA points out that, because the new reproductive techniques are medical procedures performed by physicians, the states bear the primary responsibility for regulating their quality, safety, recordkeeping, and donor-screening procedures.

Although the states have a great deal of power to protect public health, infertility treatment and research also can be regulated by the federal government through the spending power of Congress. The federal government sets health care standards with reimbursement programs such as Medicare and Medicaid. It also has a substantial impact on medical care through the regulations that control the use of federal funds for research with human subjects. Under these regulations, an institution receiving federal monies can voluntarily agree that all its research efforts—not just those that are federally funded—follow federal guidelines. Most institutions have agreed to this.

Research on fetuses, pregnant women, and in vitro fertilization is governed by specific regulations adopted in the late 1970s by the U.S. Department of Health and Human Services (DHHS). Those regulations contained a provision, however, that has, in effect, removed the federal government from the funding—and reviewing—of IVF research.

The provision stated that research concerning IVF could not be supported by the DHHS unless each research proposal was reviewed by the Ethics Advisory Board (EAB) for its ethical acceptability. As noted earlier, in 1980 the EAB ceased to exist. Although a charter for a new EAB was drafted in 1988, no action has resulted.

The absence of an EAB has obliterated the path that researchers normally would follow to receive federal funding for IVF and GIFT research. As a result, most such research is privately funded, with no federal overview. As the OTA pointed out in its infertility report, "No uniform protocol for IVF exists. Further, the technique never went through a formal or regulatory research stage in the United States to demonstrate either safety or efficacy, in large part due to the lack of Federal direction and Federal funding."

IVF CLINICS—THE CURRENT SCENE

In its study on infertility, the OTA found that IVF and GIFT procedures are being performed in a variety of settings, from single-doctor offices to large university medical complexes. Most IVF clinics are non-profit entities associated with a university or a hospital, and most offer a range of therapies for female infertility in addition to IVF. The centers are located chiefly in areas with large populations. Older centers known for their good results have waiting lists of one to two years. This, along with the increasing number of young couples who find themselves infertile and are financially able and eager to resolve their dilemma, has helped to encourage the proliferation of new IVF clinics.

Most IVF clinics are supported by patient fees. According to the OTA, patient fees make up 80 to 100 percent of a clinic's income. The cost of infertility treatment depends on the severity of the cause. A complete diagnostic workup of both partners can cost $2,500 to $3,000, although not all cases of infertility require such extensive evaluation. Each embryo transfer costs between $4,000 and $7,000. Additional costs can be substantial in time spent away from work and, if the treatment center is located some distance away, travel and hotel expenses. The OTA estimates that a couple experiencing severe female infertility could easily spend over $20,000 for four embryo transfers, which might give the couple a 50 percent chance of taking home a baby.

In general, private health insurance plans cover about 70 percent of the cost of infertility treatments other than IVF techniques. Insurers have been reluctant to include IVF treatment in their health coverage because each implantation attempt is expensive and because they feel no upper limit has been set on the number of attempts. Although IVF per se has been excluded, reimbursement for some of the expensive procedures that are part of it, such as laparoscopy, generally is included.

The OTA does not believe that the increase in the number of clinics, the resulting competition, or any improvements in success rates are likely to reduce fees in the near future. That observation is based on the knowledge that most of the laboratory and surgical techniques used in IVF are common hospital procedures with standardized charges. The additional fees charged for the fertilization and incubation process and, on occasion, for research, generally are not a large proportion of the total charges.

The 1982 National Survey of Family Growth (NSFG) revealed that more white women than black women use infertility services, despite the fact that infertility is one and a half times greater among black couples. Infertility services are used more frequently by women who are better educated, married, and have a high income. The NSFG found that some 200,000 women with primary infertility had never sought help. Researchers believe the reason may lie in the scarcity of low-cost therapy for infertility. In the mid-1980s only 21 percent of physicians treating infertility accepted Medicaid patients and only 6 percent varied their fees for low-income patients.

Current costs for infertility treatment are so substantial that they place infertility care beyond the reach of low-income couples, and they represent a sizable investment for middle-income couples. For couples with before-tax annual incomes under $20,000, the cost per stage of treatment would range from 6 to 62 percent of their annual income. Infertility therapy could consume 2 to 23 percent of the annual income of couples whose incomes range between $20,000 and $35,000. For those with incomes over $35,000, treatment costs represent between 1 and 12 percent of annual income.

Those figures apply only to couples who have health insurance. As the OTA emphasizes, they underestimate the burden of infertility costs on couples whose incomes are in the low to middle range, many of whom are either not insured or underinsured.

RESEARCH NEEDS

Observers believe that current treatments for infertility would produce better results and new ones would be developed, particularly for male infertility, if an EAB existed to lend guidance on the ethical issues associated with such research. The OTA estimates that if federal funding were made available as many as 100 projects would be proposed. Examples of the areas needing study include:

• Embryos today are chosen for implantation largely by their appearance. More exact information on the determinants of a healthy embryo may increase the chance of a successful pregnancy.

• All human embryos may not survive when frozen for future use. Researchers would like to devise methods to enhance embryo survivability.

• There is no definite formula for calculating the number of sperm to be placed near the egg for a successful fertilization in IVF and GIFT. The development of more precise data may improve fertilization rates.

• To improve chances of conception using frozen sperm, more must be known about cryopreservation, the true effectiveness of frozen semen, and methods for improving that effectiveness.

• Sperm deficiencies are evident in 30 to 40 percent of infertile couples, yet few methods exist for determining healthy sperm, and not enough is known about the basic process of sperm movement through the female reproductive tract.

• Not all causes of male infertility are known, thus limiting the treatments available.

CONCLUSION

Infertility appears to be on the rise in the United States among young couples, and increasing numbers of affected couples of all ages are seeking solutions. Since 1978 the techniques of in vitro fertilization and its variations have been added to the more traditional surgical and medical treatments for this disorder. In the swiftness of their development and proliferation, however, the new therapies for reproductive failure have raised public and professional concerns about quality control, public oversight, and advertising.

IVF moved quickly from experimental to clinical status. The number of clinics offering IVF has grown from 10 to 165 in five years. Because the avenue to federal funding for this research has been blocked by the

38

SCIENCE AND BABIES

demise of the mandated EAB, there has been no federal oversight of this research and its clinical application. Although minimum standards for IVF centers have been promulgated by professional societies, centers are not obligated to follow them, and there is no mechanism for overseeing clinic claims or quality.

As a result, the claims made by individual clinics about their success rates are open to manipulation. There are clinics that have not produced a single baby, and there are centers using success rates taken from other clinics. Those seeking IVF therapy and physicians making referrals have few means to evaluate the quality of an IVF clinic or the accuracy of its claims. The need for standards, licensing, and government regulation is beginning to be discussed in public forums. Whether a new EAB will be chartered is unknown. In the meantime, licensing embryo laboratories and providing basic information on IVF clinic performance are important first steps toward protecting consumers.

ACKNOWLEDGMENTS

Chapter 2 was based in part on presentations by Robert G. Edwards and Lorraine V. Klerman.

REFERENCES

American Fertility Society. 1984. Minimal standards for programs of in vitro fertilization. Fertility and Sterility. 41:13.
American Fertility Society. 1988. Minimal standards for gamete intrafallopian transfer (GIFT). Fertility and Sterility. 50:20.
Balmaceda, J.P., C. Gastaldi, J. Remohi, C. Borrero, T. Ord, and R. Asch. 1988. Tubal embryo transfer as a treatment for infertility due to male factor. Fertility and Sterility. 50:476-479.
Blackwell, R.E., B.R. Carr, R.J. Chang, A.H. DeCherney, A.F. Haney, W.R. Keye, Jr., R.W. Rebar, J.A. Rock, Z. Rosenwaks, M.M. Seibel, and M.R. Soules. 1987. Are we exploiting the infertile couple? Fertility and Sterility. 48:735-736.
Centers for Disease Control. 1988. Semen banking, organ and tissue transplantation, and HIV antibody testing. Morbidity and Mortality Weekly Report. 37:57-58, 63.
D'Adamo, A.F., Jr. 1987. Reproductive technologies: the two sides of the glass jar. In Women & Health. Binghamton, N.Y.: The Haworth Press. 13:9-30.
Edwards, R.G. 1986. Current clinical, scientific and ethical situation of human in vitro fertilization. I.J.M.S. 155:275-286.
Ellis, G.B. 1988. Testimony at the Hearing on Consumer Protection Issues Involving In Vitro Fertilization Clinics, before House Subcommittee on Regulation and Business Opportunities. Washington, D.C. June 1.
Harkness, C. 1987. The Infertility Book. San Francisco: Volcano Press.

Infertility—Medical and Social Choices. 1988. Washington, D.C.: U.S. Congress, Office of Technology Assessment, OTA-BA-358.

Jansen, R.P.S., J.C. Anderson, and P.D. Sutherland. 1988. Nonoperative embryo transfer to the fallopian tube. New England Journal of Medicine. 319:288-291.

Jones, H.W., Jr. 1986. Status of basic external human fertilization. Paper presented at Institute of Medicine planning meeting, Washington, D.C. May 9.

McShane, P.M. 1987. In vitro fertilization, GIFT and related technologies—hope in a test tube. In *Women & Health.* Binghamton, N.Y.: The Haworth Press. 13:31-46.

Marrs, R.P. 1988. Testimony at the Hearing on Consumer Protection Issues Involving In Vitro Fertilization Clinics, before the House Subcommittee on Regulation and Business Opportunities, Washington, D.C. June 1.

Mascola, L., and M.E. Guinan. 1986. Screening to reduce transmission of sexually transmitted diseases in semen used for artificial insemination. New England Journal of Medicine. 314:1354-1359.

Matson, P.L., D.G. Blackledge, P.A. Richardson, S.R. Turner, J.M. Yovich, and J.L. Yovic. 1987. The role of gamete intrafallopian transfer (GIFT) in the treatment of oligospermic infertility. Fertility and Sterility. 48:608-615.

Medical Research International, the Society of Assisted Reproductive Technology of the American Fertility Society. 1989. In vitro fertilization/embryo transfer in the United States: 1987 results from the national IVF/ET registry. Fertility and Sterility. 50:13-19.

Mosher, W.D. 1987. Infertility: why business is booming. American Demographics. July:42-43.

National Center for Health Statistics, W.D. Mosher and W.F. Pratt. 1985. Fecundity and infertility in the United States, 1965-82. Vital and Health Statistics, U.S. Department of Health and Human Services, Washington, D.C. February 11:1-7.

National Institutes of Health. 1989. Sex can cause more than AIDS. Healthline. August:3-4.

N.Y. Times. 1988. Pressure to regulate in vitro fertilization grows as demand rises. July 28. B-7.

Peterson, E.P., N.J. Alexander, and K.S. Moghissi. 1988. A.I.D. and AIDS—too close for comfort. Fertility and Sterility. 49:209-210.

Raymond, C.A. 1988. In vitro fertilization enters stormy adolescence as experts debate the odds. Journal of the American Medical Association. 259:464-469.

Schinfeld, J.S., T.E. Elkins, C.M. Strong. 1986. Ethical considerations in the management of infertility. Journal of Reproductive Medicine. 31:1038-1042.

Seibel, M.M. 1988. A new era in reproductive technology: in vitro fertilization, gamete intrafallopian transfer, and donated gametes and embryos. New England Journal of Medicine. 318:828-834.

Sherman, J.K. 1987. Frozen semen: efficiency in artificial insemination and advantage in testing for acquired immune deficiency syndrome. Fertility and Sterility. 47:19-21.

Steptoe, P.C., R.G. Edwards, D.E. Walters. 1986. Observations on 767 clinical pregnancies and 500 births after human in vitro fertilization. Human Reproduction. 1:89-94.

Wallach, E.E. 1988. Testimony at the Hearing on Consumer Protection Issues Involving In Vitro Fertilization Clinics, before the House Subcommittee on Regulation and Business Opportunities, Washington, D.C. June 1.

Wassarman, P.M. 1988. Fertilization in mammals. Scientific American. December: 78-84.

Wyden, R. 1989. Opening remarks and testimony at the Hearing on Consumer Protection Issues Involving In Vitro Fertilization Clinics, before the House Subcommittee on Regulation, Business Opportunities, and Energy, Washington, D.C. March 9.

3
Contraception
Having a Healthy Baby at the Right Time

Contraception has been practiced in some form since ancient times. The Petri Papyrus of Egypt, which dates to 1850 B.C., carries a prescription for a pessary made of sodium carbonate and honey. Another Egyptian formula of that time was crocodile dung mixed with a pastelike material. In the mid-1700s, Casanova recommended capping the cervix with half a lemon, from which the juice had been removed. Condoms date back to ancient Egypt and China, where men used sheaths made from animal membranes or oiled silk. The word "condom" was first used in England and may derive from the name of a Dr. Condom, who supposedly made a protective sheath for King Charles II to stem his number of illegitimate children.

In the early 1900s, a movement to make contraceptives and family planning services available to U.S. women got under way with Margaret Sanger's first birth control clinics. The synthesis of two orally active progestogens in 1951, followed by the successful testing of these steroids as oral contraceptives, began a campaign for widespread access to birth control in the 1960s described by some observers as a "contraceptive revolution."

The development of the birth control pill, plus a renewed interest in the IUD, came at a time when rapid population growth was being perceived as a threat to the global environment and to the economic and social health of many countries, particularly those in the Third World.

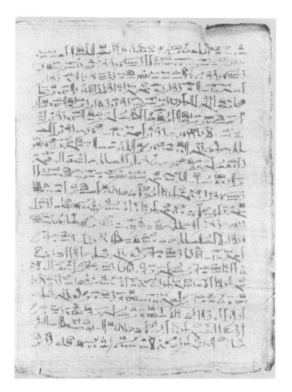

This scrap of papyrus is a prescription written in 1550 BC for a medicated tampon to prevent conception. Soaked in a mixture of honey and the fermented tips of acacia bush, the tampon was used as a vaginal suppository. Stewed acacia leaves produce lactic acid, an effective spermicidal ingredient also used in contraceptive ointments in the 1940s and 1950s. The papyrus was discovered by George Ebers in Luxor in 1873. Credit: National Library of Medicine

In the United States, the increasing number of women entering the work force created new demand for the control that contraception could give over one's reproductive life. Stirred by these concerns, governments for the first time began to fund research on population and contraceptive development.

The success of the pill encouraged the pharmaceutical industry to become vigorously involved in developing new contraceptives. By the mid-1970s, 13 pharmaceutical companies, 9 of them in the United States, were active in the field, and observers predicted that many new approaches to contraception would soon be available. Expectations included a pill for men and a vaccine against pregnancy for women. As recently as 1982 the congressional Office of Technology Assessment estimated that by the end of this century more than 20 new or significantly improved technologies for contraception would be available.

Although these expectations were based on the number of studies under way, interest and funding soon declined and the predictions have yet to become realities. In fact, the opposite has occurred. Writing in *Family Planning Perspectives* in early 1988, Richard Lincoln and Lisa Kaeser of the Alan Guttmacher Institute observed:

> If in the 1960s we saw the birth of a contraceptive revolution, then in the 1980s we are witnessing the failure of that revolution and the reversal of many of its hard-won gains. In the United States, where the pill and the modern IUD were first developed, contraceptive methods are disappearing faster than new ones can be introduced.

Until very recently IUDs were almost unavailable to women in the United States; today only two models, the copper-releasing ParaGard and the progestogen-releasing Progestasert, are marketed. Injectable contraceptives, such as Depo-Provera, which are used in practically every country of the world, are not allowed here. Several new birth control pills on the market in Europe cannot be prescribed in the United States, although they are considered safer. The pills contain new progestins that are thought to cause fewer adverse effects on the cardiovascular system than the older progestins. RU 486, an abortifacient and menstrual inducer, is being marketed in France and China, but at present there is no plan to seek the approval of the Food and Drug Administration (FDA) for use in this country. Lincoln and Kaeser state that clinical research on new contraceptive methods is practically at a standstill in this country; only two American pharmaceutical companies, Ortho and Wyeth, are doing any contraceptive research at all.

In the United States, as in many countries, women begin having intercourse at a younger age than did women living earlier in this century. At the same time, many wish to have small families. Observes Dr. Malcolm Potts, president of Family Health International:

> The median age at which U.S. women have their last wanted child is 26.9 years, and 75 percent of all women have all the children they want by age 30. Even a contraceptive method with an annual failure rate of one percent that is used from age 30 to age 45 will leave one woman in seven with an unintended pregnancy.

At first it may seem that there are many birth control choices in the United States, but close examination reveals the opposite. Oral contraceptives are used chiefly by women under age 30 because physicians are anxious about the cardiovascular side effects of the pill among women over age 35. Furthermore, misinformation about the possible health effects of the pill discourages many young women and teenagers from using it. Also because of side effects, IUDs today are being prescribed only for women in mutually monogamous relationships who have at least one child. Barrier methods such as the condom and diaphragm are less effective than the IUD or the pill and are unattractive to many couples.

Because their choices for truly safe and effective contraceptives are limited, American women often have long intervals during which they are not protected against the possibility of pregnancy. As a result, over 50 percent of them have unintended pregnancies, and thus the United States has a higher rate of abortions than most other industrialized countries.

WHY THE DECLINE IN CONTRACEPTIVE DEVELOPMENT?

Many factors played a role in the decline of contraceptive research and development. Some were economic; others were political and social. Research on reproduction and contraception is expensive and complex and takes years. Because reproduction is species specific, much of the experimental work must be conducted with humans, a pursuit that requires high-priced and sometimes unavailable liability insurance. In addition, some side effects, such as the thromboembolic effects of the pill, may develop only after extensive use and cannot be found beforehand, making the contraceptive business extremely vulnerable to litigation.

Such risks do not encourage pharmaceutical companies to enter the field of contraceptive development. In fact, most of the companies that once were involved in this research have left, and other companies have reduced their commitment.

Certain developments have accelerated the decline of contraceptive research, particularly research on entirely new contraceptive methods. The most harmful developments have been the proliferation of product liability suits and the sharp rise in liability insurance premiums. Other negative factors include the lack of both public and private financial support and a time-consuming FDA approval process.

The Lawsuit Proliferation

In 1982 the National Survey of Family Growth (NSFG) found that the IUD was the fifth most popular reversible form of contraception in the United States, with just over 2 million women using it. A few years later the three most commonly used IUDs were taken off the market.

The Dalkon Shield, made by A.H. Robins Company, was removed from the market when a flood of damage suits were filed against it beginning in 1975. The design of the Dalkon Shield, which went on the market in 1971, before FDA approval of medical devices was required, was clearly associated with an increased risk of pelvic infection, subsequent infertility, and, in some cases, death. The Robins Company knew of the potential hazards but denied them; other IUDs, which are free of the Dalkon Shield defects, have been suspect ever since.

Until recently, G.D. Searle and Company made the only copper IUDs available in the United States. Copper-carrying devices have a lower pregnancy rate than noncopper ones and their association with pelvic inflammatory disease has been low. Nevertheless, Searle faces about 350 claims for damages and is appealing a jury verdict that awarded a plaintiff in Minnesota over $8.1 million. (The jury found Searle negligent in advertising and labeling its Cu-7 IUD.) Searle's cost of defending four lawsuits initiated in 1985, which it won, totaled $1.5 million.

By the mid-1980s, both Searle and Ortho Pharmaceutical Corporation decided to stop selling IUDs. Ortho based its decision on the fact that its market for the Lippes Loop was being eroded by an overall decline in IUD sales and by the increasing market share of the copper IUDs. Although its copper IUDs were popular, Searle decided to stop marketing them in North America. It continues to sell IUDs in 18 other countries, where it has encountered very few lawsuits. Searle decided to leave the U.S. market because of the high cost of defending itself in liability suits and the difficulty of obtaining liability insurance. Currently, two IUDs are available in the United States: the Progestasert, made by Alza Corporation, and the copper-wrapped ParaGard, distributed by GynoPharma, Inc., under license from the Population Council.

Carl Djerassi, a contraceptive expert at Stanford University, described other negative effects of liability litigation when he wrote:

> In 1980, several pharmaceutical companies claimed to have had more product liability claims for oral contraceptives than for all other drugs combined, notwithstanding that probably no group of currently used prescription drugs has been tested clinically as thoroughly as these steroids. It is not even the fact that few of these suits are won by the plaintiffs. It is just that the financial, human, and administrative costs of pursuing them are so high that few companies wish to expose themselves to such waste.

Djerassi claimed that although most of the active ingredients in the birth control pills being used are off patent, generic equivalents are just beginning to appear on the market, no new companies are entering the field, and, in contrast to other drugs no longer under patent, the price of oral contraceptives is continually increasing.

In 1985 the Upjohn Company announced it was phasing out its fertility research program. As its reasons the company cited the increase in adverse litigation, the long approval process, and rising insurance costs. Some observers suspect that hostility from antiabortion activists influenced Upjohn as much as anything else. Although Upjohn is no longer studying prostaglandins for their contraceptive value, the company continues to investigate the compounds as possible treatments for ulcers and cardiovascular disease.

The increase in the number of lawsuits was not the only significant upward trend in the 1980s. Jury awards became so large they made headlines. Similarly, the cost of defending malpractice and product liability lawsuits rose. A study by the Institute of Civil Justice at the Rand Corporation revealed that between 1982 and 1985 there was a 15 percent annual increase in the cost of defending both malpractice claims and product liability suits. The cost for defending more routine automobile claims rose only 6.3 percent annually.

Changes in the Legal Rules

During the past two decades, major modifications were made in the rules governing liability lawsuits, reports Deborah Hensler of the Institute of Civil Justice. The locality rule for malpractice suits was overturned, and new bases for bringing claims, setting damages, and measuring loss were established. Negligence was no longer necessary as a basis for a product lawsuit; instead, manufacturers could be held to new and strict concepts of liability. In many jurisdictions the statute of limitations was relaxed for injuries that might take more years to develop, and, as with malpractice, new ways of determining loss were introduced. In describing the result, Dr. Hensler notes, "There have been numerous small, substantive changes in the law that most people agree have increased grounds for plaintiffs to bring claims, increased their chances of being successful, and increased their chances, if they are successful, of winning large awards."

Also during the past two decades important changes in procedural rules boosted the number of successful claims and drove up the amount of jury awards. For example, the rules governing "discovery" permitted a greater exchange of the information on which a lawsuit was built, an important factor in litigation that uses massive amounts of technical and medical data. Dr. Hensler notes that the proportion of large law firms has increased and more of them are specializing. In fact, some law firms concentrate on cases involving only particular products. In addition, attorneys today use computer technology to build data bases of the discovery documents developed for particular cases, and these data bases are being shared among lawyers nationwide.

Two objectives of the tort liability system are to make restitution to injured people and to deter bad behavior. But studies have found that people with modest losses are overcompensated for their economic damages, people with large losses are undercompensated, and those with very large losses are severely undercompensated. As a method of making amends, the tort system is costly and not very equitable.

How well does the system deter negligent behavior? Dr. Hensler believes that more attention is being paid by the medical profession to quality of care. Manufacturers of products, particularly risky products, seem to agree that their general level of consciousness about safety is higher than it was in the past. But the price for such consciousness raising also appears high and the method is not efficient.

Unfortunately for manufacturers, medical care personnel, and institutions that might look to litigation outcomes for performance guidelines, information produced by the legal system is not always clear or consistent. Court decisions vary from state to state and, within states, from jury to jury. It would be very hard to determine from reading just the appellate cases what the standard of a particular type of care should be.

And the tort system may be overdeterring, causing beneficial services and products to be removed from the market. The withdrawal of most types of IUDs is one example. Dr. Hensler reports that surveys in 1983 and 1987 by the American College of Obstetricians and Gynecologists showed a sharp increase in the percentage of clinicians who said they were limiting their practice with regard to high-risk patients. The survey found that some specialists also no longer provide certain obstetrical services because of concerns about liability.

The tort liability system and the regulatory system that has been built in this country do not always coordinate well. Many providers of medical care and products find themselves caught between the two. For example, FDA rules can be used as a basis for making judgments in tort liability suits while in the same lawsuits FDA rules are not allowed as a defense. There are controversies over these rules, and some efforts toward changing them are being made. Dr. Hensler has noted, however, that opposition to change is strong, in part because of concern for patient and consumer safety and in part because of bureaucratic reluctance.

The chilling, unplanned-for effect of court decisions on medical care and on the availability of safe contraceptives is an indirect cost of these unsystematic and poorly understood changes in the tort system. Some observers believe it is time to focus on such consequences of the system and how they affect all who participate in the health care process.

The Increased Cost of Insurance

Consumers who are injured by a product may expect remuneration from the manufacturer, either through the courts or directly. Those costs, which can be extremely high, are covered by professional and product liability insurance. Conventional liability insurance from commercial insurers has become either impossible to obtain or very expensive in recent years for many products and services, particularly for contraceptives. Large corporations in the field, such as Ortho, can afford liability insurance or can set aside profits for self-insurance. But although they may refine current products, they are deterred from developing new contraceptives. Public sector organizations, such as universities and nonprofit groups like the Population Council, which have been responsible for much of the contraceptive development and some of the field's more innovative research, do not have the funds to pay for commercial insurance or to insure themselves.

For smaller contraceptive developers, testing on human subjects has almost stopped because the availability of insurance to cover the testing is either not dependable from year to year or not available at all. But the cost and availability of liability insurance may not be related to the volume of lawsuits or to the cost of defending them. Some observers feel that the paradox is tied instead to interest rates and profitability: Liability claims rose at a time when interest rates on invested premiums declined, reducing the insurer's profit margin. When interest rates were high, critics say, insurers were interested in writing product liability insurance; when the rates dropped, insurers compensated by canceling policies held by contraceptive developers.

Others in the field take a different point of view, saying that liability insurance for contraceptives is not feasible to underwrite because insurance companies simply cannot assess the liability exposure of a particular contraceptive product. Contraceptives appear to be an example of a class of mass-marketed products that have the latent capability of causing disease and injuries among some users. Such products are viewed as having a highly uncertain but potentially enormous liability risk. Whatever the reasons, the high cost of insurance has had a distinct negative effect on contraceptive research and the development of new methods.

Individual states and the U.S. Congress are considering a range of bills that would reform both the tort system and liability insurance laws. Whether these reforms are passed and whether contraceptives will be covered by such legislation seems unlikely in the near future.

The Funding Gap

Funding for contraceptive development by the pharmaceutical industry and by governments worldwide peaked in 1972 at $74.3 million. It dropped substantially three years later, and by 1983 spending leveled off at just under $57 million, spread over 384 research projects involving 70 variations of potential contraceptives. That amounted to just under $150,000 per project. Ortho says that bringing a new contraceptive method from the laboratory to the market costs the company about $125 million and the process generally takes 10 years, or $1.25 million per year for one type of contraceptive. Modifications of existing drugs require less time and money.

The low level of funding has had several results. Most obvious is that the focus of research has not been on the expensive process of discovering new methods of contraception that would be either safer or more acceptable to people for whom present methods are not an option. Instead, efforts have concentrated on the less expensive process of modifying existing drugs. Consequently, most of the contraceptives currently available here and abroad are based on the progestogens synthesized almost 40 years ago, including injectable steroids such as Depo-Provera, steroid-releasing implantable capsules, and steroid-releasing vaginal rings.

Skimpy funding slows the development of new contraceptives by limiting the number of drug combinations or formulas that can be explored at a time. Lincoln and Kaeser state that the new Norplant implantable capsules could have reached the market many years earlier if more money had been available during its early years of research. Sixteen years passed before Norplant was marketed in any country.

In the United States today there is less basic research under way at universities and other nonprofit institutions than there has been since the early 1970s. At $9 million for fiscal 1989, federal funding for contraceptive research and development is extremely low. Low levels of private and government support tend to discourage young scientists from entering the field, inhibiting new discoveries and the use of new knowledge from other areas for contraceptive development.

FDA Requirements

In 1962, after the thalidomide tragedy, the FDA developed new procedures to test the safety and efficacy of drugs. Conforming to the new mandates lengthened the overall time required for drug development.

A later change that had a considerable effect on the development of contraceptives was a requirement for very stringent toxicology and carcinogenicity testing in animals for new contraceptives. For other noncontraceptive drugs, the choice of animals, usually rats and rabbits, was left to the investigating scientist, and the required lengths of the repeated-dose toxicity studies used to evaluate the cumulative effects of drugs were 2 weeks, 4 weeks, and 6 months for Phases I, II, and III, respectively.

For contraceptive drugs, however, testing requirements were made stiffer. The FDA insisted that toxicology testing be performed in rats, dogs, and monkeys and that it extend for 90 days, 1 year, and 2 years for each of the three phases. While carcinogenicity testing for other drugs consisted of 2-year rat and 18-month mouse trials, for contraceptives those tests had to be "lifetime" trials of 7 years in dogs and 10 years in monkeys.

Dr. C. Wayne Bardin, vice president of the Population Council, observes that, "In retrospect, the toxicity testing in animals correctly predicted that steroidal contraceptives were relatively free of risk compared to other drugs." But such testing, he said, "was not successful at predicting many of the rare but serious adverse effects of hormonal contraceptives, such as thromboembolism and hypertension."

Not surprisingly, the very high doses used in the animal studies produced diseases in dogs that had not been observed in humans. As a result, many contraceptive drugs were withdrawn from development on the basis of what in retrospect appears, Dr. Bardin says, to be spurious observations in animals.

In early 1988 the FDA revised its requirements for testing contraceptive steroids to conform more closely to the guidelines espoused by the World Health Organization (WHO). Today for the first time FDA requirements for testing contraceptive drugs are almost identical to the requirements for other drugs.

In its guidelines the WHO does not recommend beagle and monkey studies for contraceptive drugs because available data indicate that findings of certain cancers in these animals are not accurate predictors of such cancers in humans.

Still time-consuming and expensive, however, is the amount of documentation needed to get FDA permission for clinical trials. The annual reports on such studies must be written in substantially more detail than in the past. Other countries are also requiring increasingly detailed documentation. For large companies this means the expense of thousands of man-hours. For the smaller public sector organizations, the requirements can be almost impossible to meet; at best, the requirements add years to the process before a contraceptive can be made available to the public.

Pharmaceutical companies gain financial support for their research on both successful and unsuccessful contraceptive products from the sales of those products that do reach the market. Their profits increase with the length of time they have exclusive rights to the product while it is under patent. Until such exclusivity was extended somewhat in 1985, patent protection lasted 17 years. Under the original FDA approval process, contraceptive development in the United States took a long time, sometimes almost the entire life of the patent. With little opportunity to recoup their costs, pharmaceutical companies have had little incentive to develop new contraceptives. In 1988 Dr. Potts noted:

> By the time manufacturers bring a new formulation to the marketplace, half or more of the 17-year patent life may be over, so there is little commercial incentive for expensive postmarketing surveillance. Either we need to make premarket testing cheaper and postmarketing surveillance obligatory or we need to find federal money to support the necessary postmarketing studies.

The clinical trials required by the FDA generally are two years long and seldom utilize more than 2,500 women. These clinical trials and the animal tests performed before the drugs are approved for marketing cannot detect the infrequent but serious side effects that may appear only after long-term use in a large number of women. The WHO has suggested that the health of contraceptive steroid users might be better protected if more emphasis were placed on postmarketing surveillance and less on animal testing. Organized postmarketing surveillance programs may prove to be more consistent and accurate in documenting any long-term adverse effects of contraceptives.

The WHO, Family Health International, and the Population Council have a joint postmarketing surveillance program under way in seven countries to learn about any possible rare events associated with long-term use of Norplant. The program will follow some 8,000 Norplant users and 8,000 controls for 5 years. This approach also has been adopted for in vitro fertilization; the National Institutes of Health has contracted with Medical Research International to follow 13,000 women treated with IVF and similar procedures.

The lack of adequate funding, the lengthy FDA approval process, the fluctuating availability of insurance coverage, the increase in the number of lawsuits, and the changes in the legal rules have had a chilling effect on contraceptive development. There is concern that the range of contraceptive methods will remain narrow and that very few contraceptive methods—perhaps none—will gain widespread acceptance among the large number of women of different ages and varying cultural backgrounds, in the United States and throughout the world, who do not now use contraceptives.

THE NEED FOR BETTER CONTRACEPTION

To Prevent Abortions

In the many developed countries where small families are desired, abortion rates decline with the increased use of contraceptives. Jacqueline Darroch Forrest of the Alan Guttmacher Institute recently observed:

> While recognizing that peoples of the world hold differing judgments regarding the moral and ethical dimensions of contraception and abortion, there is little disagreement that contraception is almost always a more efficient and safer way to limit births than is abortion.

In industrialized countries that maintain data on unplanned pregnancies and abortions, it is clear that abortion rates mirror the number of unintended pregnancies. The number of unplanned pregnancies and, subsequently, the number of abortions are lower in countries where effective contraceptive methods are widely used.

U.S. women have more unintended pregnancies and abortions than do women in other industrialized nations. When the reproductive and contraceptive behavior of women aged 15 to 44 in the United States and 19 other similarly westernized countries was studied in the early 1980s, the levels of sexual activity were found to be quite similar. U.S. women, however, were found to use contraceptives at a much lower rate and, in turn, had much higher rates of pregnancy, abortion, and childbearing, particularly in their teens and early 20s. Included with the United States in this study were the countries of Western Europe plus Canada, Australia, and New Zealand.

Among countries worldwide that keep accurate abortion statistics, the abortion rate for women ranges from 5.6 per 1,000 women in the Netherlands to 70.5 in Yugoslavia. The U.S. abortion rate is 28.5, placing it in the middle of the range, with Singapore and East Germany. The average U.S. couple wants 1.25 children but winds up having 1.8 and also, on average, approximately one abortion.

In the United States in 1982, the most recent year for which there are data from the NSFG, some 6.1 million women became pregnant. Of those pregnancies, more than half were unintended, including the 1.6 million abortions and a third of the 3.7 million births.

To Slow Population Growth

The 1968 publication of Paul Ehrlich's book *The Population Bomb* alerted this country and the world to the dangers of out-of-control population growth. By 1970 U.S. birth rates dropped to replacement levels, an event announced by Walter Cronkite during his evening news program. The nation appeared to heave a sigh of relief and turned its attention to other matters. U.S. support boosted family planning programs in many of the most populous developing countries during the 1970s; the programs were just beginning to demonstrate an impact when the effort was weakened in the 1980s by changes in U.S. administrative policies. If the world population continues to multiply at the current rate, in the 100 years between 1923 and 2023 it will have quadrupled.

Eleven countries are responsible for 70 percent of the world's increase in population: Bangladesh, Brazil, China, India, Indonesia, Japan, Mexico, Nigeria, Pakistan, the Soviet Union, and the United States. Carl Djerassi states that only 3 of the 11—Japan, the Soviet Union, and the United States—have acceptable population growth rates. Djerassi points out that although these three can be described as having their population growth under control, in two of them control is achieved largely through the use of abortion. At 11 million abortions each year among a population of 275 million, the Soviet Union has the highest per capita abortion rate in the world. Japan, which still does not permit the use of oral contraceptives, has an estimated 528,000 abortions per year in a country of 120 million people. The United States has the highest teenage abortion rate of any industrialized country. Says Dr. Djerassi: "Here are three countries that presumably have the situation under control but . . . there are segments of the population that are very ill-served."

In the next century, 90 percent of the increase in world population will occur in the poorer developing countries, with African nations expanding at the greatest rate. *Time* recently reported that in the poorest countries growth rates are outstripping the national ability to provide housing, fuel, and food. The effects of burgeoning populations have become so grim that some environmentalists are urging that the current population growth be cut by one-half during the next 10 years. The World Fertility and Contraceptive Prevalence Surveys of the Agency for International Development show that couples in Third World countries want fewer children. They are prevented from doing so because they do not have access to family planning programs. Dr. Malcom Potts believes expenditures for Third World family planning programs could be doubled and still not meet all the need for contraception.

In many nations the increased use of contraceptives parallels not only a decrease in population growth but also an increase in the quality of life. Quality of life is determined by the human suffering index developed by Population Crisis Committee researchers. This index measures such essential human needs as income, inflation, demand for new jobs, urban population pressures, infant mortality, nutrition, clean water, energy use, adult literacy, and personal freedom.

To Improve Maternal and Child Health

Contraceptive methods do more than avert the dangers posed by undesired population growth. At the individual level, men and women wish to limit the size of their families, to delay starting a family, or to space the births of children in order to enhance their own personal and economic opportunities and to provide their children with good health and a stable home. Unwanted pregnancies put these goals out of reach for many people as well as threaten the health of mothers and children.

The World Fertility Surveys show that in almost all developing countries more than half the women want to stop having children or desire to space the births of their children. In many of these nations, very high rates of maternal and infant mortality and morbidity can be attributed to illegal abortions, to births less than a year apart, and to childbearing at very young or older ages. In Egypt, for example, half the annual national mortality rate is attributed to women over age 30 who died having a third, fourth, fifth, or later child.

In any country, regardless of its development status, as the use of contraceptives increases, the rates for both infant and maternal mortality decrease. Family planning influences the health and lives of women and children in important ways: It averts the need for abortion. It permits young women to avoid pregnancy until they are more emotionally and economically prepared to take care of a child. It permits women to space their children to allow their bodies to recover between births, an important consideration when a mother is not well nourished. A woman who has fewer children is less likely to have a low birthweight infant or a pregnancy complication.

To Increase the Choice of Effective Methods

For a variety of reasons, not all of which are known, women and couples may not use contraception even when it is available in their community or they may choose a method that is not very effective. Techniques such as periodic abstinence, douching, or withdrawal are associated with high failure rates but are still commonly used. About 4.6 million women worldwide used such methods during 1987. Such techniques may be selected over more effective approaches because they do not cost anything, require little planning ahead, or have no side effects. Or they are used because a couple does not have access to a better alternative. Women who are poor or young use contraceptives less consistently. Worldwide each year there are 10 to 30 million pregnancies because of contraceptive failure, and many of these pregnancies are voluntarily terminated.

Contraceptive choices are affected not only by the needs of the individual but also by male and female perceptions of the safety and effectiveness of a particular method. A 1985 survey by the Gallup organization of women's attitudes toward contraception revealed that a substantial majority of U.S. women are seriously misinformed about the safety and efficacy of the methods currently available. They view birth control as being less effective and as having more side effects than is true. Women are especially misinformed about oral contraceptives. Research reports regarding the pill and breast cancer have worsened the situation by demonstrating conflicting results, confusing physicians as well as the public.

The Gallup survey found that 76 percent of U.S. women believed that there were substantial risks associated with using oral contraceptives. The findings also revealed that not many Americans realize that women still die in childbirth and that the overall U.S. maternal mortality rate, 14 per 100,000 live births, is almost three times the rate of pill-related deaths. A survey of middle-class urban women in eight developing countries found that 50 to 75 percent had similar misconceptions about the pill's health effects.

Birth control pills appear to be extremely safe for young women. In the United States, for a woman under age 35 who smokes fewer than 15 cigarettes a day, it is safer to use the pill than to deliver a baby. Oral contraceptives also reduce the risk of endometrial cancer, cysts and cancer of the ovaries, benign breast tumors, pelvic inflammatory disease, and ectopic pregnancies. The benefits of the pill in cancer protection equal or outweigh the cardiovascular risks.

Any contraceptive method that includes steroid compounds has the potential to produce side effects that can range from minor to serious. Any side effects must be evaluated by the woman and her physician or family planning person. It was proposed in 1970 that both the serious and minor side effects of birth control pills might be related to the amount of estrogen in the pill. Since then pills with lower doses of both the estrogen and progestogen components have been marketed.

The first oral contraceptive contained 150 micrograms of an estrogen and 10 milligrams of a progestogen. Today the commonly used pills contain much lower doses: 30 to 50 micrograms of an estrogen and 1 milligrams or less of a progestogen. In recent years the relationship between progestogen dosage and a rise in blood lipid levels has been given increased attention; researchers hope that reducing the dose will lessen this effect.

Dr. Djerassi has suggested that it also may be necessary to find ways to communicate to the public that "safe" cannot mean absolutely safe. "Absolute safety is a chimera," he cautioned, "as is true in every other aspect of life."

To Increase Acceptability and Accessibility

For voluntary family planning to succeed, contraceptive options must be effective, inexpensive, and available. There must be an ample choice of methods to meet the individual needs of people who are of different ages, who come from different ethnic and educational backgrounds, who live in diverse socioeconomic conditions, and who often have limited access to health services.

Prospective contraceptive users include women at different stages in their reproductive lives; each stage has different contraceptive requirements. The birth control needs for individuals or for couples change as their lives change. The diaphragm that was acceptable when a man and woman were dating may be too interruptive when they are married. The health status of either partner may dictate a switch from the pill to the condom or an IUD. For instance, if the woman is a heavy smoker and she and her partner are monogamous, she may want to use an IUD rather than the pill. At another point in their lives, after having the number of children they want, a couple may decide on sterilization.

Studies show that intercourse is not something that most young women in the United States just beginning to date "plan" to have. Yet birth control methods require at least some planning, if only to buy a tube of spermicide or a contraceptive sponge. Because the pill is not directly associated with coitus, young women appear to be more comfortable using it. However, getting a prescription for the pill does require a visit to a clinic or private physician, and using it effectively requires a minimum of consistent effort.

In this country the pattern of contraceptive use among unmarried women of reproductive age changes over time. The NSFG showed that just under 47 percent of women aged 15 to 44 were protected against pregnancy when they had premarital intercourse for the first time. The leading method was the condom, followed by the pill and withdrawal.

During the months after first intercourse, more and more of the young women who practiced contraception began to use the pill and fewer depended on withdrawal and condoms. At the 12-month mark, almost 70 percent were using the pill, 11 percent were protected by condom use, and fewer than 2 percent depended on withdrawal. By that time, too, more women, 17 percent, had discovered and were using other methods of contraception.

Researchers in family planning emphasize that many variables—demographic, psychosocial, and community—affect the use of contraceptives in the early days of sexual activity. Research that includes all these variables is necessary before effective intervention strategies can be devised to prevent early unintended pregnancies. Analyses based on the NSFG estimate that at any one time there are 3.3 million fertile, sexually active women at risk of unintended pregnancy who do not use any method of contraception.

As Mahmoud F. Fathalla of the World Health Organization put it, there will always be a "yes" group of highly motivated people who want to use contraception and a "no" group of those idealogically opposed to the concept. But in between there is a large group for whom the availability of inexpensive and convenient methods could tip the balance toward their using contraception.

A contraceptive may be highly effective, inexpensive or free of cost, and readily available and still not be used, because the technology is unattractive to that particular population. The acceptability of a contraceptive method depends a great deal on how it fits into the perceptions, culture, or life-style of the prospective user.

Social scientists have observed that modern contraceptives have certain inherent attributes, such as the sex of the user, the relationship to coitus, the need to handle the genitalia, or the need for repeated applications. Susan C.M. Scrimshaw of the University of California at Los Angeles School of Public Health explains that each of these inherent attributes elicits different responses in different cultures. For example, cultures in which women are not allowed to cook for their families during episodes of vaginal bleeding (as in India) are less accepting of the IUD, which is associated with increased bleeding. Dr. Scrimshaw found that women in Spanish Harlem prefer sterilization as a birth control method because they had to confess that to their priest only once. Some men and women will not use diaphragms, condoms, or cervical caps because they dislike handling their genitals.

In addition to the inherent attributes, a set of "perceived" attributes tend to grow around each contraceptive method. Dr. Scrimshaw says:

> While these attributes, such as the notion in Ecuador that the birth control pill "eats the red blood cells," are not true, they nevertheless affect acceptability. If people believe them, they are likely to reject the method just as they would for a culturally or individually undesirable inherent attribute.

It is also possible to have culturally acceptable methods and to deliver them in such a way that they are used only minimally. Research has shown that factors such as the type of clinic, its location and hours, the attitudes or other characteristics of the staff, the tone of staff-to-patient interaction, and communication with the community all may have an impact on the acceptability of a program. The cost of a contraceptive method also is a major factor in its acceptability. Cultural customs also can play an important role. Six months after birth control pills were supplied directly to women in Iran, only 12 precent of the women were still taking them. When the pills were distributed to the husbands to give to their wives, 90 percent of the women continued to take them after six months.

To make contraceptive methods attractive and acceptable to varied ethnic groups, it is sensible to fit the technology to the people, rather than the people to the technology. Although additional basic research is needed to develop more contraceptives, those in existence could be utilized more fully if they were made acceptable to more populations. Dr. Scrimshaw believes acceptability can be enhanced by utilizing information from the behavioral and social sciences:

> It is difficult to measure behavior accurately and consistently and even more difficult to predict it. But when new technologies and programs are launched without any such measurements, not only can costly errors occur, but it may be years before it is even clear the programs aren't working.

It is important to note that not all contraceptives are distributed via clinics. Many are successfully marketed to the general public by being sold over the counter in pharmacies and other retail outlets, including the smallest village shops. In some countries oral contraceptives are vigorously advertised; in many communities they are widely available without a prescription. In some areas the pill is available from village women who have been trained to screen prospective users for contraindications. Subsidizing the price of contraceptives also has made them more acceptable and cost-effective.

No single method can meet the needs of one woman or one couple, much less the needs of an entire population, particularly in a heterogeneous country such as the United States. For contraceptives to be used effectively, a "contraceptive supermarket" is necessary, Dr. Djerassi says, "from which people can pick and choose, because there is no such thing as an ideal contraceptive" for all populations.

HINDERING CONTRACEPTIVE USE

Why does the United States differ so markedly from other industrialized countries in behaviors associated with reproductive health? Thirteen percent of sexually active unmarried women of childbearing age in this country do not practice birth control. Why is this so? In its study of unintended pregnancy, contraceptive practice, and family planning services in

20 industrialized nations, researchers from the Alan Guttmacher Institute noted these contrasts between the United States and similar countries:

• In other countries contraceptive care is integrated into primary health services and is available at locations that are many, familiar, and convenient. This is not true in the United States.

• In many countries where the use of effective methods is high and pregnancy and abortion rates are low, contraceptive care is delivered chiefly by family physicians rather than by specialists. The family physicians are especially likely to prescribe oral contraceptives. In the United States obstetricians and gynecologists provide most contraceptive care.

• Family planning clinics in other countries are designed to serve mostly first-time contraceptive users and other groups who may require special counseling. They frequently offer evening or weekend hours, female personnel, and a variety of contraceptive choices. In contrast, U.S. clinics are meant to provide free or low-cost services to people too poor to obtain contraceptive care from private physicians. In the United States the choice of a caregiver is determined by the patient's financial state; in other countries the determinant is the patient's needs.

• The choice of contraceptives in the United States is narrower than in other countries. A number of improved or entirely new methods, including injectable contraceptives and lower-dose formulations of the pill, are not available.

• In most of the countries studied, but not in the United States, contraceptives are free or inexpensive.

• Information about contraception and sexuality is widely disseminated in some other countries through advertising, publicity, education, or the distribution of literature from pharmacists. In countries where the condom is widely advertised, for example, it tends to be more widely used.

Two other major barriers hinder U.S. women from using contraceptives. One is the widespread absence of information, especially among the young and not well educated, about the dangers of getting pregnant and about contraception. The other is the negative attitude held by a sizable proportion of women toward the most effective contraceptive methods. Furthermore, in other nations contraceptive information and advertising are disseminated through the media, including national television. Although the conventional thinking in the United States is that most Americans do not want sex education in the schools and do not want to have contraceptives advertised on national television, recent nationwide opinion polls show the reverse to be true. A 1985 Gallup poll found that three-fourths of Americans want sex education to be taught and that they thought it should be done before high school.

A 1987 survey by the Louis Harris organization found that most Americans have no religious or moral objections to family planning. Six out of 10 questioned approved of advertising contraceptives on television. Seventy-two percent, including 73 percent of Catholics and 60 percent of Evangelicals, said contraceptive advertising would not offend people like themselves. The Harris poll also reported that 76 percent of Americans thought "if young people saw that TV stars they admire use birth control," they would be more likely to use it themselves. A smaller survey of 800 adults conducted about the same time by NBC and the *Wall Street Journal* found that 79 percent of respondents approved of contraceptive advertising.

Favorable attitudes are a prerequisite for the use of birth control. Better dissemination of information would help eliminate the barrier to contraceptive use caused by negative attitudes toward the pill and the IUD, according to the Gallup poll and a 1987 Guttmacher study of women at risk for unintended pregnancy. Those surveys found that women avoid using the pill and IUD, the most effective methods, because they fear potential health risks. Women also underestimate the efficacy of these methods.

Their concern is understandable. In recent years there have been many news articles about the lawsuits over damage caused by the Dalkon Shield IUD. Most cases of pelvic inflammatory disease (PID) associated with the IUD are related to exposure to sexually transmitted diseases. In addition, insertion of an IUD may introduce bacteria into the genital area, which is why so many of the infections appear early. Because PID can lead to infertility, IUD use today is limited to women who already have at least one child and are in a mutually monogamous, stable relationship.

A 35-member American Medical Association Diagnostic and Therapeutic Technology Assessment panel recently pronounced the Progestasert and the ParaGard—the two IUDs available in the United States—safe and effective when users are carefully selected. The opinion of the panel is important because an IUD fills an important niche in birth control: It offers effective contraception for the mature woman for whom oral contraceptives may no longer be ideal.

Studies of oral contraceptive use show that the pill is much safer than

U.S. women believe. The mortality risk has dropped with the increased use of modern-day pills and the discouragement of pill use among women over age 35 who smoke. As Malcolm Potts says, "If analysis of the health impact of oral contraceptive use is limited to cardiovascular risks and to the prevention of ovarian and uterine cancer, the good and bad effects virtually cancel each other out."

It is certain that the pill has no important adverse or beneficial effects on breast cancer. However, more information is needed about the pill's relationship with that very small but tragic group of women who develop breast cancer before age 45. Several recent, small epidemiological studies suggest a link between pill use at an early age (before age 20 or the first pregnancy) and early breast cancer. Because of inconsistencies among these studies, the FDA believes the new evidence is not clear cut enough to warrant changing the prescribing rules for oral contraceptives. Nevertheless, the possible association between the pill and breast cancer in young women is an important concern, and a broad investigation is under way at the Institute of Medicine.

Regular and accurate updates on the safety and efficacy of contraceptives are important in keeping women apprised of contraceptive facts. A flow of accurate information will help women of all ages and educational backgrounds find a contraceptive that is right for them.

CONCLUSION

Contraceptives are not new, yet their development and use in the United States are impeded by substantial obstacles. Contraceptive development is markedly hindered by a lack of funds, the proliferation of lawsuits, exorbitant jury awards, and an absence of liability insurance for contraceptive manufacturers. Many men and women in this country are badly informed about birth control and about the true effectiveness and health risks of the methods that are available. Half the pregnancies in this country are unintended, and the United States has one of the highest rates of abortion and teenage pregnancy among industrialized countries.

Better contraception is needed in the United States—and throughout the world—to broaden the choice of effective approaches so that men and women of diverse ethnic backgrounds can find contraceptives with which they are comfortable. The experience of other nations suggests that to reduce the number of unintended pregnancies and abortions in this country, particularly among teenagers, we must make contraceptives more easily available and we must be more vigorous in our dissemination of information about birth control and family planning.

Birth Control Methods Available in the United States Today and Their Effectiveness

Sterilization for men and women is the leading method of contraception in the United States; it is safe and 100 percent effective. In general, it is not reversible, although sophisticated new sterilization methods are being developed that may make it possible to reverse the procedure in some cases.

Birth control pills are 95 to 99 percent effective and need less planning than other substantially effective methods such as the diaphragm and condom. They do not require any handling of the genitals nor do they interrupt foreplay. Modern-day pills that combine low doses of estrogens and progestogen have fewer adverse effects on the cardiovascular system than the pills of 30 years ago. A mini-pill with no estrogen is available for women who are breastfeeding or over age 35 and smoke. The combination pill is not recommended for lactating women. Although oral contraceptives may have undesirable side effects for some individuals, they protect against cancers of the ovaries and uterus and against excessive menstrual bleeding.

Intrauterine devices are 98 to 99 percent effective. Of the two types currently available, the copper-releasing Paragard needs to be changed every 4 years, the progestogen-releasing Progestasert once a year. Because IUDs have been associated with an increased risk of pelvic inflammatory disease, which can cause infertility, the makers of IUDs recommend that they be used only by women who have had at least one child and are in a stable, mutually monogamous relationship. After an IUD is inserted by a trained health care provider, it requires only an occasional check by the wearer to ensure that it is still in place.

The *condom* is growing in popularity because it is readily available and offers good protection against sexually transmitted diseases, particularly those brands coated with a spermicide. Spermicide creams or foams can be added to the inside and outside of a condom for extra protection. The failure rate ranges from 3 to 15 percent, with failure often ascribed to careless use. Because condoms can leak or break, experts recommend that the female partner use a spermicide foam as extra protection. Condoms have no adverse side effects, although the spermicide coating may cause an allergic reaction in some men and women.

The *diaphragm* produces few side effects; it can cause urinary tract infections, and some women may be allergic to the spermicidal cream or jelly that must be used with it. Its failure rates range from 2 to 20 percent, with most failures arising from improper or inconsistent use. If used consistently, however, experts believe the diaphragm is highly effective. In addition, it offers some protection against sexually transmitted diseases. The diaphragm must be fitted by a health care provider, and the fit must be checked by a health professional every few years or after childbearing or a substantial weight change.

Norplant, a contraceptive implant, steadily diffuses a low dose of the progestin levonorgestrel directly into the bloodstream. Norplant is more effective than oral contraceptives and is free of estrogen. It can cause menstrual irregulatory, but thus far has produced no serious side effects. Norplant capsules are surgically inserted under the skin of the arm by a trained health care provider and protect against pregnancy for 5 years. The capsules should be removed at the end of that time because they become less effective. They can be removed earlier if desired. The United States will be the thirteenth country to approve Norplant for use; the method is in clinical trials in some four dozen other countries.

Sponges, foams, creams, jellies, and vaginal suppositories are easier to obtain because they can be bought in a drugstore and are easy to use. They do have a failure rate of 3 to 21 percent. Researchers do not know if this relatively high failure rate is due to inconsistent use or to inadequacies inherent in the methods. These vaginal methods protect against pregnancy by inactivating the sperm. To be effective, the sponge must be kept in place for at least 6 hours after intercourse. To avoid possible side effects, it should be removed after 24 hours. Because the same active ingredient, nonoxynol-9, is used in all of these products, if a woman is allergic to one product, she cannot use any of them.

The *cervical cap* resembles a small diaphragm. It is filled with a spermicidal foam or jelly and placed over the cervix. As effective as a diaphragm, it has an added advantage in that it can be inserted several days before intercourse and can be left in longer afterward. If left in place too long, the cervical cap begins to have an odor. Some users report that the cap, which is smaller than a diaphragm, allows more sexual pleasure; it also may be a better choice for women with recurring urinary tract infections. Accurate placement requires practice. Since receiving FDA approval in 1988, cervical caps have been manufactured in the United States; they are available chiefly in large population centers, often through women's health groups.

Birth Control Methods on the Horizon for the United States

A number of fertility-regulating methods may be available in the United States in the next 10 to 15 years if sufficient funding is made available. When funding is in short supply, research efforts must be cut back. As a result, development can be stretched out over many more years, delaying the availability of new methods.

Two types of *vaginal rings* that release steroids into the bloodstream via the vaginal epithelium are being studied by the Population Council and the World Health Organization. One releases a combination of estrogen and progestogen and is worn for 3 weeks; the other, which releases the progestogen levonorgestrel, is worn continuously for 3 months and is designed for women who are breastfeeding. The rings are self-inserted. Although they can cause irregular bleeding, they have fewer side effects than the pill. Their effectiveness appears to be high, but studies are not yet complete.

Biodegradable pellets of norethindrone or levonorgestrel, implanted just under the skin, are effective for 12 to 24 months. They appear to be highly effective and are now undergoing clinical trials.

A *female condom* is being developed. Like the male condom, it would protect against sexually transmitted diseases, would be readily available, and has no apparent side effects. Used with a lubricant, it is inserted by the woman.

Transdermal delivery of hormones is a method that releases contraceptive steroids slowly into the circulatory system through the skin via a patch worn on the body. In the system currently being studied in the United States, a new skin patch is applied each week for 3 weeks, followed by a week without a patch to allow menstruation to occur.

Birth Control Methods Not Available in the United States

Injectable contraceptives—Depo-Provera and Norigest—appear to be highly effective and are convenient. Currently, both injectables are available in the United States for menstrual problems and endometriosis but not for birth control. Depending on the dosage, the slow-release injection into a muscle can be given every 3 or 6 months. The larger, longer-lasting dose may produce more side effects, such as headaches, weight gain, depression, and irregular bleeding. Injections of progestogen alone can cause irregular menstrual bleeding, but another formulation that adds estrogen appears to produce regular bleeding patterns in most women. Widely used in many countries, injectables are still being studied for contraceptive use in the United States.

The *CuFix 390* intrauterine device is a string of hanging copper rings, a design that lessens the chance of pain, bleeding, and expulsion that is sometimes associated with IUDs. It has performed well in early trials in other countries, but because of the product liability climate in the United States, its manufacturers might not seek marketing approval here.

Abortifacients and menstrual inducers fill a major need in current birth control technology because they can be used a few days or weeks after unprotected intercourse to induce menstruation. The most studied is the antiprogestin, mifepristone, known as RU 486, which is available in France and China. A dose of 600 milligrams of mifepristone followed by 1 to 10 milligrams of prostaglandin brings on menstruation in over 95 percent of the women who use it. The use of RU 486 requires medical supervision. Although any attempt to market this drug in the United States is expected to lead to protests from antiabortion segments, the laws of many countries permit "menstrual therapy" even when surgically induced abortion is not allowed. Although new methods of postcoital contraception will certainly be opposed by some members of society, in many parts of the world an inexpensive self-administered menstrual inducer is expected to receive broad acceptance.

ACKNOWLEDGMENTS

Chapter 3 was based in part on presentations by Carl Djerassi, Deborah Hensler, Malcom Potts, and Susan Scrimshaw.

REFERENCES

American College of Obstetricians and Gynecologists. 1985. Gallup poll shows what public knows and thinks about birth control. Press release, March 6. Washington, D.C.

Atkinson, L.E., R. Lincoln, and J.D. Forrest. 1985. Worldwide trends in funding for contraceptive research and evaluation. Family Planning Perspectives. 17(5):196-207.

Atkinson, L.E., R. Lincoln, and J.D. Forrest. 1986. The next contraceptive revolution. Family Planning Perspectives. 18(1):19-26.

Bardin, C.W. 1987. Public sector contraceptive development: history, problems, and prospects for the future. Technology in Society. 9:289-305.

Cushner, I.M. 1986. Reproductive technologies: new choices, new hopes, new dilemmas. Family Planning Perspectives. 18(3):129-132.

Diagnostic and Therapeutic Technology Assessment panel. 1989. Questions and answers: intrauterine devices. Journal of the American Medical Association. 261(14):2127-2130.

Djerassi, C. 1987. Contraception in the year 2001. In *Contraception in the Year 2001*, edited by P.A. van Keep, K.E. Davis, and D. de Weid. Amsterdam: Elsevier Science Publishers.

Djerassi, C. 1989. The bitter pill. Science. 245:356-361.

Ehrlich, P.R. 1968. *The Population Bomb*. New York: Ballantine Books, Inc.

Family Health International. 1987. Women's perceptions of the safety of the pill: a survey in eight developing countries. Co-ordinator: Gary S. Grubb. Journal of Biosocial Sciences. 19:313-321.

Fathalla, M.F. 1988. New contraceptive methods and reproductive health. In *Proceedings of the Conference on Demographic and Programmatic Consequences of Contraceptive Innovations*, edited by S. Segal, A. Tsui, and S. Rogers. New York: Plenum Press.

Forrest, J.D. 1986. The end of IUD marketing in the United States: what does it mean for American women? Family Planning Perspectives. 18(2):52-55.

Forrest, J.D. 1987. Unintended pregnancy among American women. Family Planning Perspectives. 19(2):76-77.

Forrest, J.D. 1988. U.S. women's contraceptive attitudes and practice: how have they changed in the 1980s? Family Planning Perspectives. 20(3):112-118.

Forrest, J.D., and S.K. Henshaw. 1988. Effects of new contraceptive methods on abortion utilization. In *Proceedings of the Conference on Demographic and Programmatic Consequences of Contraceptive Innovations*, edited by S. Segal, A. Tsui, and S. Rogers. New York: Plenum Press.

Grimes, D.A. 1986. Reversible contraception for the 1980s. Journal of the American Medical Association. 255(1):69-74.

Alan Guttmacher Institute. 1985. Risk of developing primary infertility is at least twice as high for IUD users as for never-users. Family Planning Perspectives. 17(4):182-183.

Alan Guttmacher Institute. 1987. Poll says most people accept family planning, approve of condom ads. Family Planning Perspectives. 19(2):79.

Hatcher, R.A., D. Kowal, F. Guest, et al. 1989. *Contraceptive Technology: International Edition*. Atlanta: Printed Matter, Inc.

Henshaw, S.K. 1987. Characteristics of U.S. woman having abortions, 1982-1983. Family Planning Perspectives. 19(1):5-9.

Henshaw, S.K. 1988. The characteristics and prior contraceptive use of U.S. abortion patients. Family Planning Perspectives. 20(4):158-168.

Jones, E.F., J.D. Forrest, S.K. Henshaw, J. Silverman, and A. Torres. 1988. Unintended pregnancy, contraceptive practice and family planning services in developed countries. Family Planning Perspectives. 20(2):53-67.

Kolata, G. 1989. For those concerned with pill risk, a look at the choices. N.Y. Times. January 12, B-10.

Lincoln, R., and L. Kaeser. 1988. Whatever happened to the contraceptive revolution? Family Planning Perspectives. 20(1):20-24.

Mosher, W.D., and C.A. Bachrach. 1987. First premarital contraceptive use: United States, 1960-82. Studies in Family Planning. 18(2):83-95.

PATH and PIACT. 1987. FDA may follow WHO guidelines for contraceptive steroid testing. Outlook. December, 9-10.

PATH and PIACT. 1988. FDA confirms new requirements for steroid testing. Outlook. March, 10.

PATH and PIACT. 1988. More contraceptive choices likely by end of century. Outlook. 6(4):2-8.

Population Crisis Committee. 1985. Issues in contraceptive development. Population, No. 15 May. Washington, D.C.

Potts, M. 1988. Birth control methods in the United States. Family Planning Perspectives. 20(6):288-297.

Rosoff, J.I. 1988. Not just teenagers. Family Planning Perspectives. 20(2):52-67.

Silverman, J., A. Torres, and J.D. Forrest. 1987. Barriers to contraceptive services. Family Planning Perspectives. 19(3):94-102.

Special Programme of Research, Development, and Research Training in Human Reproduction. 1987. *Guidelines for the Toxicological and Clinical Assessment and Postregistration Surveillance of Steroidal Contraceptive Drugs.* Geneva: World Health Organization.

Skuy, P. 1976. A history of contraception: how far have we really come? Canadian Pharmaceutical Journal. 109(11):3/335-5/337.

Toufexis, A. 1989. Too many mouths. Time. January 2, 48-50.

4

The Dilemma of Teenage Parenthood

Teenage pregnancy and childbearing have for some years been regarded as difficult and grave problems for the United States. Although policies and programs have been developed to reduce the incidence of children having children, their combined impact has been minimal, and the rates of adolescent pregnancy and childbearing remain high. As the Center for Population Options noted in 1988, a cycle of poverty often begins with an unintended adolescent pregnancy. Teenage pregnancies do not occur in a vacuum. Too often they are the product of economic disadvantage and inadequate educational systems, of poor housing, family instability, and the emotional deprivation associated with it. Because the children of teenage mothers have an even slimmer chance of escaping these conditions, they, too, may become adolescent parents.

The reality of almost 1 million teenage pregnancies a year demonstrates that this country's social and economic systems are failing a substantial proportion of our young citizens and, in doing so, are helping to perpetuate and enlarge the number of poor and badly educated men and women.

This chapter outlines the extent of the dilemma and examines how the United States compares with other industrialized countries in levels of teenage pregnancy, births, and abortions. It discusses the economic and social costs of adolescent childbearing on young parents and their children and on the nation. Some promising new intervention programs to prevent teenage pregnancy are reviewed, and suggestions for research on additional solutions are made. Biomedical research on the onset of puberty may provide some solutions, but the majority of the answers must come from the social and behavioral sciences.

THE SCOPE OF THE PROBLEM

In the United States each year approximately 1 out of every 10 young women between the ages of 15 and 19 becomes pregnant, a ratio that has changed little since 1973. According to the National Center for Health Statistics, in 1985 16.6 of every 1,000 girls aged 14 and younger and 109.8 of every 1,000 teenagers between ages 15 and 19 became pregnant.

The 1986 Alan Guttmacher Institute study of teenage pregnancy in industrialized countries demonstrates that the rates of adolescent pregnancy, childbearing, and abortion in the United States outstrip those of other similarly developed nations, including Canada, England and Wales, Sweden, the Netherlands, and France. In England and Wales the pregnancy rate among girls 14 and younger is 3 per 1,000; for 19 year olds, it is 86 per 1,000.

Although the pregnancy rate for black adolescents in the United States is considerably higher than the rate for white teens, this factor is not significant enough to explain the disparity between the United States and other industrialized nations. The pregnancy rate for U.S. white adolescents alone is twice as high as the rate for teenage pregnancies in Canada, the country closest to the United States in its proportion of teen pregnancies.

This disparity is all the more puzzling when viewed against the fact that, according to the Guttmacher study, U.S. teenagers are no more sexually active than their peers in similar countries. The frequency of abortion and pregnancy in the United States cannot be accounted for by a greater frequency of sexual activity.

Despite efforts at the federal and state levels and by many private agencies to reduce the number of pregnancies among the young, the percentage of U.S. teenagers who become pregnant has not changed much in the past 16 years. Researchers at the Guttmacher Institute estimate that in 1987 there were more than 1 million pregnancies among adolescents and most of them were unintended. About half the adolescents who become pregnant give birth and about half have abortions. The number of spontaneous abortions, or miscarriages, is not known, but if it were possible to record such occurrences, Dr. James Trussell, of Princeton

University, believes the total number of teenage pregnancies would rise by 10 to 15 percent.

PRECURSORS OF TEENAGE PREGNANCY

Lack of Contraceptive Use

Why does the United States differ so markedly in its levels of adolescent pregnancy, childbirth, and abortion? In reviewing data on the United States, Sweden, Canada, England and Wales, France, and the Netherlands, Dr. Trussell declares:

> The main reason for higher pregnancy rates in the United States is that American adolescents are less likely to use contraceptives regularly, or use them less effectively, than those from the other five countries. Further, among contraceptive users, smaller proportions of U.S. teenagers rely on the most effective methods, particularly the pill.

Contraceptive services and supplies are widely available and either inexpensive or free in the Netherlands, England and Wales, and Sweden. In France contraceptive services are less accessible, but the situation is improving. In Canada contraceptive services and information for teenagers are not always readily available, and nonprescription contraceptives are not covered by the national medical insurance system. In the United States a network of clinics makes services available to adolescents in most communities, but because many of the clinics were developed to serve the poor, they have a negative image and are avoided by many teenagers who consider them "welfare" clinics.

For teens who do not use clinic services, the alternative is to seek contraceptive care from a private physician. Some 30 percent of sexually active teens use private physicians for contraceptive care. But the costs of doctor visits and contraceptive supplies are often beyond the reach of many adolescents. Moreover, a substantial percentage of physicians who provide reproductive health services will not reduce their fees or accept Medicaid, making them largely inaccessible to low-income women. In general, Medicaid does not cover poor single people who do not have children or are not pregnant, poor married couples, and people whose incomes are just above the poverty levels used as Medicaid standards.

Many American teens do not have a family doctor, and many fear that a private doctor would be unwilling to provide contraceptive services to a minor or would require parental permission before doing so. Surveys of physicians show this perception to be generally accurate for pediatricians and family doctors. Few obstetricians and gynecologists, on the other hand, would refuse contraceptive care for teenagers.

Failure to use contraceptives is only part of the teenage pregnancy problem. Other forces have an important impact on whether adolescents become sexually active, whether they use contraceptives or become pregnant, and whether they terminate their pregnancies or bear a child. Each teenager is influenced by the circumstances of that particular time and environment and by her view of herself and her world.

Early Onset of Puberty and Delayed Marriage

One factor that increases the probability of a teenager becoming sexually active—and pregnant—is the fact that in industrialized countries young people reach puberty earlier and marry later, a trend that began around the 1820s. Instead of the two- or three-year time span between menarche and marriage that was usual in earlier generations, today a girl may have her first menstrual period at age 10, generally does not complete high school until she is 18, and may not marry until she is in her 20s. As Dr. Daniel Federman of the Harvard Medical School has noted: "It is this window of time within which the events we are discussing occur and for which social policy needs to be considered."

Dr. Malcolm Potts adds that "Teenage pregnancy is the kind of cruel paradox that biology and modern living play on us: in the very century when the duration of education has risen, the age of puberty has fallen dramatically."

According to Dr. Federman, the persons at greatest risk of pregnancy during this long interval between menarche and marriage are girls 15 and younger who come from poor, probably single-parent families and who are just beginning sexual activity. When adolescent girls begin to have intercourse, the frequency is generally unpredictable. A girl may not be willing and intercourse may be forced on her. Some observers feel that the ability to think logically may not be sufficiently developed at such an early age and that girls may not recognize that they are making a choice and that their choice may lead to pregnancy. However, the National Research Council Panel on Adolescent Pregnancy and Childbearing pointed out that in other countries even very young sexually active teenagers can learn to use contraceptives effectively.

To become sexually active, in essence, means the teenager makes a decision, Dr. Federman says. In some studies of adolescents, having sex has been linked with other risk-taking behaviors, such as smoking, drinking, or using illicit drugs, which some teens associate with becoming an adult. If they adopt one behavior, they are likely to adopt the others. Dr. Federman sees a difference, however. He believes that for adolescents the drive to behave reproductively can be more powerful than the drive to smoke or drink or take illicit drugs. "From my point of view, for a teenager the issue of having sex is a 'when' question, not so often a 'whether' question, as are the other decisions," Dr. Federman says.

Poverty

Poverty appears to play a major role in adolescent pregnancies. Many of the factors believed to lead to early sexual experience and pregnancy are characteristic of poverty: low-quality education, a negative perception of the future, limited employment opportunities, fatherless families, and feelings of helplessness and alienation. Children who grow up with few or no financial or familial resources may not realize how their dreams for education, marriage and a family, or a job can be hindered by early childbearing. Or they may feel they have no choices.

With inadequate basic skills, poor employment prospects, and few role models who have managed to break out of poverty, it is not surprising that many teenagers see no reason to postpone pregnancy.

Lack of Educational Goals

A strong association exists between early sexual experience and low intellectual ability, academic achievement, and a lack of educational goals. Researchers have found that many young women are below grade level in school at the time they become pregnant; others had already dropped out of school. Girls who are interested in getting an education, who score high on intelligence tests, and who are doing well in school are less likely to become sexually active at a young age. These findings may partially reflect individual ambition, regardless of family background, but much of it quite probably reflects cultural or family aspirations.

Religious Involvement

Studies show that adolescent girls are more likely to be sexually active if they are not regular church goers and if they state that religion is not very important to them. More important than any particular religious affiliation, these studies found, is the tendency to be devout and concerned about religious teachings and customs. Some observers postulate that religious teenagers may be more traditional and less inclined toward risk taking in other aspects of their behavior. In addition, the important family and social contacts in their lives may be supportive of traditional behavior.

Family Relationships

The National Research Council (NRC) panel discovered that, in general, the effect of parental relationships and communication between parent and child on teenage sexual activity may be small. Studies reveal that the parents' role in sex education is relatively minor. The panel reported:

> First, in many cases, less parent-child communication takes place than is commonly assumed; second, such communication, whether to provide information or to prescribe behavior, may not be fully heard by the child; and third, communication about sexual behavior frequently does not occur until after initiation of sexual activity.

Similarly, studies of the effect of parental supervision on teenage sexual experiences have demonstrated conflicting findings. One study showed that more supervision was associated with less sexual activity; other studies found no relationship between more supervision and adolescent sexual behavior.

Some aspects of families do have an impact. If a mother's first sexual and childbearing experiences occurred in her teens, it is probable her daughter's will as well. Girls whose families are not intact or who come from a home headed by a woman are more apt to have sexual experiences at an early age. Researchers also found that in large families the oldest child probably becomes sexually active by the time younger siblings reach adolescence, thereby providing a role model for such behavior.

When *Washington Post* investigative reporter Leon Dash researched his series on teenage pregnancy, he interviewed the members of six families begun by an adolescent pregnancy. The families were characterized not only by poverty, instability, and closely spaced births but also by a lack of affection between parents and between parents and children. Although they cannot possibly represent all families started by a teen pregnancy, their lives and words provided a glimpse of some of the reasons adolescents become pregnant. One of the teenagers Dash interviewed told him:

When girls get pregnant, it's either because they want something to hold on to that they can call their own or because of the circumstances at home. Because their mother doesn't pamper them the way they want to be pampered or they really don't have anyone to go to or talk to or call their own. Some of them do it because they resent their parents.

Peer Pressure

The influence of a teenager's peers is often cited by observers as the single most important factor affecting the initiation of sex among young men and women. But the NRC panel cautioned that peer influence may be overrated, particularly among white males and blacks of both sexes. Teenage behavior is affected as much by what they *think* their friends believe and do as by what actually occurs.

Some studies indicate that white girls may be most vulnerable to peer influences, particularly the attitudes of their closest male friends, and that peer pressure among black boys and girls seems to be relatively minor. On the other hand, after 17 months of interviewing and closely observing black adolescents and their families, Dash found that peer pressures definitely helped to encourage teens to become pregnant. Dash lived among and studied adolescents in the Washington Highlands section of Washington, D.C. Among those families, who originally were from the rural south, being sexually active, getting pregnant, and having a baby were important markers of attractiveness and of becoming an adult. Girls who still were virgins in their mid-teens were ridiculed and teased by friends and siblings. Dash wrote:

> In time it became clear that for many girls in the poverty-striken community of Washington Highlands, a baby is a tangible achievement in an otherwise dreary and empty future. It is one way of announcing: I *am* a woman. For many boys in Washington Highlands the birth of a baby represents an identical rite of passage. The boy is saying: I *am* a man.

WHAT DETERMINES CONTRACEPTIVE USE?

The National Survey of Family Growth found that fewer than half the sexually active adolescent girls who responded to the 1982 survey reported using a contraceptive the first time they had intercourse. Other research shows similar low rates of contraceptive use. In the 1976 National Survey of Young Women, 58 percent of young unmarried women who did not use a contraceptive method said they thought they could not conceive. Of the remainder, one of five said they had not expected to have intercourse. When intercourse is still a new experience, Dr. James Trussell says, not anticipating it is an even bigger factor in adolescents' failure to use contraceptives. In a 1979 study of the reasons sexually active teens did not use contraceptives, 87 percent of the young women surveyed said they did not expect to have sex.

Age

Age is an important factor in whether or not a girl is protected by a contraceptive when she first begins to have intercourse. It is also a factor in the type of method used. The older a girl is, the likelier she is to use a medical method, most often the pill. Among boys, age appears to have little effect on whether or not they use a contraceptive the first time they have intercourse.

Educational Goals

Besides helping delay sexual behavior, educational aspirations affect contraceptive decisions. Girls with clear educational goals who are doing well in school are more likely to use contraception. Similarly, the adolescent offspring of well-educated parents are more apt to use contraceptives consistently. Black girls with clear educational goals are even more likely than white girls or other black teenagers to use effective birth control.

Sex Education

Adults commonly assume that, if young people know how their bodies work and know about pregnancy and contraception, they will be more likely to seek family planning services and to use contraceptives effectively. Researchers confirm this relationship, and apparently most teens today know that a girl can become pregnant if she has intercourse. But other studies as well as letters to teenage-advice columnists in the newspapers make it clear that many teens, even those aged 17 and 18, believe they cannot become pregnant the first time they have sex or if they have sex only occasionally. Researchers questioned girls about their level of sexual knowledge and found that many didn't know enough to use contraception effectively. "The level and accuracy of knowledge among teenage girls who are sexually experienced and those who are not differ very little," the NRC report concluded.

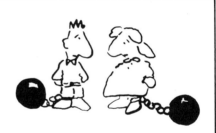

A baby is

A
LIFETIME
COMMITMENT

Are you ready for this kind of obligation?

As a pregnant teen, your priorities must change.

This advertisement is one of a series designed by college students and aimed at alerting teenagers to the consequences of pregnancy. Credit: Margaret Wehmeyer, University of Missouri at Columbia

The NRC study also found that despite what many adolescents have been taught they believe they are not at risk because they are so young. Others, girls who have avoided pregnancy successfully without birth control, believe they are immune and don't need contraceptives.

What is needed is a more thorough understanding of the connection between what adolescents know and how they behave. Douglas Kirby, in a 1989 evaluation of sex education programs and their effect on students, found that while such programs could be quite effective in increasing knowledge of conception and contraception, they apparently had little real influence on sexual behavior and contraceptive use.

For his series on teenage pregnancy, Dash interviewed adolescent parents in six families plus their mothers and other adult relatives who had become parents as teenagers. He reported that he "did not find a single instance in which procreation had been accidental on the part of *both* sexual partners. While there was some profession of ignorance about birth control among adults 40 years old and older, not one of the adolescents that I met and interviewed had been ignorant about contraception before becoming pregnant."

Although the sex education courses the teenagers had received varied in quality and thoroughness, all of the adolescents Dash interviewed were aware of birth control methods, particularly withdrawal, condoms, and the pill. They expressed a generally negative attitude toward oral contraceptives. They told Dash stories of bad things the pill could do to a woman. Whether they truly believed these tales or whether they simply did not like to use birth control is not clear. When a girl decided she wanted a baby, she would talk her boyfriend out of using condoms or withdrawal. Their statements corroborate research reports that substantial percentages of white and black adolescents fear the real or perceived side effects of birth control.

Acceptance of One's Sexual Behavior

Strongly connected with the competent use of contraceptives is the adolescent girl's acknowledgment, to herself and others, that she is sexually active. A low level of guilt and a positive attitude toward contraception also are linked with effective contraceptive use.

Stage of Development

Girls with good self-esteem who view themselves as having a certain amount of control over their lives are more apt to use contraceptives effectively. Girls who believe females should be dependent on males and who are inclined to be passive generally do not practice consistent contraception. Poor contraceptive use also is characteristic of girls who are risk takers, who find it difficult to plan ahead, or who are impulsive. These traits are also associated with boys who are poor users of contraceptives.

CONSEQUENCES OF EARLY CHILDBEARING

Knowledge of the consequences of teenage childbearing has grown as the high rate of teen pregnancy has become a fact of life in the United

States. Research findings strongly indicate that becoming a parent while an adolescent can have a negative impact on the lives of young mothers as well as on their children. The youthfulness of the mother affects her own economic, physical, and social status and that of her child. Although she may eventually improve her own life, her children may not be able to overcome the handicaps of being born to a adolescent mother.

Health Risks for Infant and Mother

Pregnant teenagers suffer more complications, miscarriages, and stillbirths than do adult women, and for girls under age 15 these dangers are intensified. Pregnant adolescents are also at greater risk of such complications as toxemia, anemia, prolonged labor, and premature labor.

Dr. Federman notes that this increased risk of complications originally was thought to be due in part to the reproductive immaturity of the very young teenager, but physical immaturity is no longer viewed as a principal factor. He says:

> If good prenatal care is given and the concerns that are appropriate for the pregnant adult woman, such as nutrition, control of anemia, control of blood pressure, and finding gestational diabetes, are extended to the teenage mother, then the medical outcomes of adolescent pregnancies are very close to the medical outcomes of married, older women in the same society.

Because nutrition directly affects the health of mother and child, babies born to teenagers, particularly poor teenagers, may be in greater danger of long-term health and developmental problems. Adolescents often have poor eating habits and these are magnified among low-income teens. Young women often begin their pregnancies with poor health habits, and they either do not know enough or cannot afford to alter their life-styles in order to produce a healthy infant. Prenatal care is especially important for pregnant adolescents, but many either do not seek care until late in their pregnancies or receive none at all. As a result, their newborns suffer disproportionately from prematurity, low birthweight, and other conditions that require extensive—and expensive—hospital care. Many of these premature infants suffer deficits that will persist throughout their lives.

About 40 percent of all teenage pregnancies are terminated by abortion. In contrast to the risks associated with early childbearing, complications from abortion occur less frequently among adolescents than among adult women, regardless of when the abortion is performed, although the earlier it is done the safer it is.

Education, Job Opportunities, and Income

Studies demonstrate that women who have children while they are in junior or senior high school are not apt to finish their education or go on to college. Teenagers who drop out of school when they are pregnant often do not return, although younger adolescents who remain at home are somewhat more likely to stay in school or return afterwards. A slightly larger proportion of older teens set up independent living arrangements, get a job, or get married and appear to be less able or willing to return to school. A study of Baltimore teenage mothers by researcher Frank. F. Furstenberg, Jr., and J. Brooks-Gunn, of the University of Pennsylvania, showed that many of the young mothers did go back to school.

Do high school dropouts catch up? According to the NRC they generally do not. Many may make notable progress in resuming their education when their children get older, but they do not catch up completely with their classmates. Young white mothers have a more difficult time than do their black peers, a fact that may reflect the existence of more extensive support systems for very young mothers in black communities or less social stigma about leaving school early.

Job opportunities and income are strongly affected by the amount of education a person receives, although that may be less true for blacks than for whites. Although family background and individual ability have some impact, receiving fewer years of education overall significantly limits both job choices and the level of attainable income. The availability of child care also influences whether a young mother can finish her education or work outside the home.

As their children grow up, women who were early childbearers enter the work force in increasing numbers. Unfortunately, their wages tend to remain at the lower end of the scale. Their incomes are not very different from those of their peers who had their children later and are working only part time.

By their late 20s and early 30s, the job status and income levels of early and later childbearers become more similar, if factors such as ability, motivation, and socioeconomic background are taken into account. However, the women who had children while in their teens tend not to marry or to have long-term solid relationships. The women who had children later are more likely to be married or in stable relationships and, despite personal low wages, are in better financial situations because they are in two-income families.

The widespread image of severe, long-term economic and social deprivation for teenage mothers and their children is exaggerated, but an examination of the long-term effects on women of adolescent childbearing shows that these women indeed are at a greater disadvantage than those who delay the birth of their first child. NRC researchers observe:

> Despite the fact that differences in work status and income between early and late childbearers diminish somewhat over time, women who enter parenthood as teenagers are at greater risk of living in poverty, both in the short and long term.

Economic Costs

Because very few teenagers who bear children are economically self-sufficient, the majority of these young women and their infants depend on public assistance programs and remain dependent longer than older families. In 1975 and 1985 studies of welfare expenditures indicated that approximately 50 percent of the total Aid to Families with Dependent Children (AFDC) subsidies went to families begun by a teenage parent.

In 1985 expenditures for the three major public assistance programs—AFDC, food stamps, and Medicaid—totaled $31.4 billion. According to estimates by researchers at the Alan Guttmacher Institute, families established as a result of an adolescent birth absorbed approximately 53 percent of that amount in 1985, or $16.65 billion. In 1987 teenage pregnancies cost the United States $19.27 billion, according to a recent report prepared by Martha R. Burt for the Center for Population Options.

Not included in these annual totals are the additional services that are more likely to be utilized by teenagers with children than by other families: housing allowances, special education programs, foster care, child protective services, and other publicly supported social services. Data on many of these costs are not available nationally.

These expenditures are high because a disproportionate percentage of adolescents who become parents are poor and must depend on public assistance for support. Not only are they more likely to need assistance, but they also tend to need greater amounts. The difficulty of finding and affording child care often prevents young mothers from entering the work force. Lack of affordable child care is a major factor in the school dropout rates of teen mothers and in their inability to take a job. Frequently, adolescent mothers are able to go to school or work only because their own mothers take care of the grand child, thus halting their educational or career opportunities. In addition, it is not easy to find employment that offers family health care benefits or a wage high enough to cover child care costs.

The majority of young mothers do not stay on AFDC. The Fursten-berg study of 300 Baltimore families begun by teenage mothers showed that the mothers were most likely to receive public assistance during the first 5 years after their child was born. After the 5-year mark, the number of young women who went off welfare increased sharply. Some would turn to public assistance again, but they left it when their circum-stances permitted. Furstenberg and his colleagues concluded that chronic or near-chronic dependence on AFDC was the exception rather than the rule among these multigenerational Baltimore families.

The Children of Teenage Mothers

What about the children of the adolescent mother? The Furstenberg study revealed that these youngsters experience a range of outcomes as they become teenagers themselves, but too often the environmental factors that led their mothers to early parenthood can have the same effect on their offspring. Dr. Daniel Federman observed that many children of adolescent parents have social and developmental handicaps that can be detected in their first years. They frequently are less healthy than the children of older married parents, their school performance is less favorable, and the daughters of teenage mothers disproportionately are very likely to become adolescent mothers themselves.

Although research evidence is not extensive, the studies that do exist indicate that the age of a mother at the birth of her child can affect the child's intelligence, as measured on standardized tests, and his or her academic achievement. In both sexes at all ages small differences in cognitive functioning appear consistently.

What accounts for these differences? As the NRC panel reported, adolescent mothers tend to be poor and less educated. As a result, their children are more apt to grow up in disadvantaged neighborhoods, to attend low-quality schools, and to experience more family stress and instability. The biggest factor is the extent and quality of their mother's education. According to one study, children's IQ scores decline by approximately one point for every year of schooling their mother does not complete.

Furstenberg's Baltimore study found that the children of teenage mothers had average scores at ages 4 and 5, but in their adolescent years their record in school was described by the researchers as dismal. Some had already dropped out of school.

In addition to problems with cognitive development, the offspring of teenage parents grow up with more social impairments, such as poor anger control, fearfulness, and feelings of inferiority. They also demonstrate mild behavior disorders, such as rebelliousness, aggression, and impulsiveness. The Furstenberg study reported that the adolescent children of teenage mothers exhibited a relatively high degree of school behavior problems and were frequently expelled. Twenty-one percent of these children had stolen something of significant value, and 28 percent had been picked up by the police for questioning. Substance abuse and early sexual activity also were common among these youngsters. Interviewing these families 20 years later, Dr. Furstenberg and his colleagues found that one-third of the adolescent daughters of the teenage mothers in the study had become pregnant before age 19.

In Volume II of *Risking the Future*, Sandra L. Hofferth, of the Urban Institute, concluded that much of the effect a teenage parent has on a child's social and intellectual development is indirect. She found, for example, that the unstable family structure that often characterizes teenage parenthood may have especially negative effects on the children as they reach adolescence.

The mothering skills of a teenage girl depend heavily on her family situation, education, the availability of support systems, her experiences, and her knowledge of childrearing. Investigators point out that the widespread assumption that teenagers automatically make poor parents is too simplistic and not supported by research. Studies in this area began in the 1980s and are not extensive, but thus far few differences have been found between the mothering styles of teenagers and older women. Adolescent mothers tend to talk less to their children, which may be related to the lower cognitive scores of their preschoolers.

Although findings so far are incomplete and not clear, it appears that the incidence of learning disabilities, delinquency, and child abuse in teenage families is related not so much to the age of the parents but to family insecurity and other socioeconomic factors. Many of the same elements that lead many teenagers to early sexual activity and early childbearing outside of marriage also have significant effects on their offspring. Poverty, the quality of the mother's education, and family size and solidity, rather than the mother's age, play the more direct negative roles in teenage families.

Research also shows that economic dependence and early childbearing outside marriage are not always repeated through the generations. A wide diversity of outcomes among the women and children is demonstrated in Furstenberg's Baltimore study. Today many of those adolescent mothers are finding routes to social and economic recovery. Of their children, some appear to be headed for productive adulthood. The recently completed 20-year follow-up of these families shows that some of the children are catching up by finishing high school or getting jobs just a little later than the children of women who delayed childbearing.

The future of the children of adolescent mothers is of considerable concern to observers who believe it is associated with early sexual experiences and pregnancy in girls and with antisocial behavior in boys.

AVERTING TEENAGE PREGNANCY

There is considerable agreement in this country about the need to reduce the incidence of adolescent pregnancy, although those who disagree with the methods to reduce it are very visible and vocal and often generate a lot of controversy. Polls by the Louis Harris organization in 1985 and 1988 demonstrated that 85 percent of Americans want sex education taught in the public schools. According to the 1985 poll, 67 percent would support laws requiring schools to establish links with family planning clinics, where teenagers could go to obtain contraceptives, and 78 percent thought television should feature birth control advertising.

Since the early 1970s, the number and types of programs aimed at helping young women and men avoid unintended pregnancies and births have increased substantially. Some programs concentrate on increasing teenagers' knowledge of human reproduction, family relationships, and decision making; some offer family planning services; and some are designed to improve youngsters' educational and job opportunities.

Sex Education Programs

Public opinion polls have consistently showed that a majority of Americans believe children should be taught about reproduction in school so they can make informed decisions about their own sexual behavior. In response, states have become more supportive of such programs. A 1982 survey of 179 major city school districts found that three-fourths provided some sex education in junior and senior high schools and two-thirds provided it in elementary school.

On the negative side, sex education courses tend to be short—fewer than 10 hours—and to concentrate on the physiology of sex. Not all students take the courses. In the elementary and junior high grades, only a small number of these classes discuss contraceptive methods. Programs in senior high school are broader, and three-fourths of them cover family planning, contraceptive methods, and abortion.

The obstacles to sex education are many. The Alan Guttmacher Institute surveyed secondary public school teachers who were entrusted with sex education courses. When asked about what they regarded as obstacles to teaching the subject, they mentioned the difficulty of changing students' ideas about sex and pregnancy, school boards with Victorian attitudes, lack of support from department heads, inadequate funding, and weak support from parents and the community, often because adults are not well informed about sexual matters.

A variety of private community-based groups, such as the YWCA, churches, the Scouts, and the Salvation Army, also sponsor sex education courses.

One of the more successful privately funded programs was a cooperative effort between the Johns Hopkins University School of Medicine and the Baltimore City Department of Education. Designed to prevent pregnancy among urban teenagers, the Self Center program served a senior high school and a junior high school that had a combined enrollment of 1,700. Many of the students were drawn from an inner-city neighborhood that contained low-cost and public housing; base-line questionnaires revealed a high level of sexual activity among the students. The program included classroom presentations; educational and counseling services provided in the schools; and educational, counseling, and medical services in a nearby storefront clinic open only to students from the two schools. A full-time social worker and nurse practitioner were available in each school and after school at the clinic. The project was unusual in that it combined services and research and used two other city schools as controls for evaluating the program.

Over a period of 3 school years, the Self Center project achieved many of its goals. It markedly improved the level of student knowledge of contraception and pregnancy risk, it significantly increased the use of clinics and of contraceptive methods among teenagers already sexually active, and it was able to draw males into its program.

Of particular interest were two results: (1) students exposed to the project for all 3 years postponed their first intercourse experience for an average of 7 months and (2) contraceptive use increased among all age groups attending Self Center programs, particularly among students who participated for 3 years. The active use of the storefront clinic and the interest in contraception were underscored when the pregnancy rates for the Self Center schools were compared with those of the two control schools. After 28 months, pregnancies in the control schools increased by 58 percent; in the Self Center schools, pregnancies dropped by 30 percent. The Johns Hopkins researchers reported:

> While the changes in the age at first intercourse are not large, they are substantial enough—in the direction of delay—to refute charges that access to such services as those provided by the program encourages early sexual activity. The program's ability to effect any further changes may well have been limited by the brevity of the project and the age of the students when they were first reached.

The average expense for this comprehensive program was $122 per student; the class lectures cost $5.56 per presentation per student; students who used all the available services cost the program about $546 each.

The Self Center was an experimental program that ran from 1981 to 1984; although it no longer exists, some Baltimore schools now have school-based clinics. The clinics do not provide contraceptives, but they do refer students to local family planning centers.

The evaluation component of the Self Center program clearly demonstrated the effect of a comprehensive pregnancy prevention program on behavior. There is considerable anxiety among some segments of U.S. society that such programs, or their components, might encourage earlier sexual activity among adolescents. Others question the effectiveness of family life/sex education programs in promoting responsible contraception among teenagers who already are sexually active.

The Johns Hopkins pregnancy prevention program provides strong evidence that a comprehensive service can help adolescents to postpone sexual activity and, if they are already sexually experienced, to avoid pregnancy. In addition, this program demonstrates that such a service does not lead to increased sexual activity.

Other studies also have found no link between sex education courses and an increase in sexual activity. Although not as clear-cut in their methodology as the Self Center program, these studies do indicate that teenagers who were already sexually active are somewhat more apt to use contraception and are less likely to become pregnant if they receive some sex education.

According to Dr. Federman, the expense of preventing pregnancy is dwarfed by the expense of experiencing it. The costs of sex education and family life programs in particular are very low, dramatically so compared with the amount of money needed to support a teenage mother and her child for just one year. The NRC study panel on teenage pregnancy found that the federal share of supporting a young family was $18,710 in 1979 dollars. In contrast, the average per-student cost of classroom sex education lectures in the state of Illinois came to $10 a year, similar to the Baltimore cost.

The many families begun by teenage pregnancies annually cost the public billions of dollars. As noted earlier in this chapter, the United States in 1987 spent a total of $19.27 billion on these families. That figure included both administrative costs and direct payments to providers of AFDC, Medicaid, and food stamps. It did not include the costs of other publicly supported services such as foster care, housing supplements, or special education. A young woman who had a baby in 1987 and who will receive welfare for about 8 years will cost the public approximately $38,700. Delaying such births markedly reduces such public outlays.

Efforts to Promote Chastity

Many people feel that the best way to reduce the number of teenage pregnancies is to persuade adolescents not to have sexual intercourse. Reasonable people agree that sexual intercourse in the younger teen years benefits no one. The problem is determining which of the variables influencing the onset of sexual behavior are open to change. The 1981 Title XX Adolescent Family Life Act, which replaced earlier legislation for adolescent health care and pregnancy prevention services, was designed to put added emphasis on preventing early sexual intercourse.

The goal is a sensible one; the issue is how to achieve it. In the 1981 act less emphasis was given to birth control services. Instead, the legislation sought to encourage premarital chastity by promoting strong family values; it also encouraged the use of adoption as an alternative to teenage childrearing.

In *Risking the Future* the NRC study panel reported that critics of the family life program declare its approach is inappropriately moralistic. The American Civil Liberties Union has brought suit against Title XX on the basis that it represents a mixing of church and state.

Although some observers believe sex education programs that promote personal responsibility may help some adolescents postpone intercourse, others feel that a large proportion of teenagers will continue to become sexually active. Experienced researchers are not hopeful that changes in sexual behavior will occur, especially in an environment in which sex and sexiness are portrayed as important attributes in television shows, movies, popular magazines, newspapers, and advertising. Researchers at the Guttmacher Institute note:

> American teenagers seem to have inherited the worst of all possible worlds regarding their exposure to messages about sex: Movies, music, radio and TV tell them that sex is romantic, exciting, titillating; premarital sex and cohabitation are visible ways of life among the adults they see and hear about. . . .Yet, at the same time, young people get the message good girls should say no. Almost nothing that they see or hear about sex informs them about contraception or the importance of avoiding pregnancy.

The Guttmacher study concluded by noting that European countries concentrate on preventing teen *pregnancy* and the United States concentrates on preventing teen *sex*, and that is why Europe is more successful in reducing the number of adolescent pregnancies.

Improving Access to Contraception

For the sexually active teenager who wants to use birth control, family planning services are available in almost every large community. Providers include state and city public health departments, school-based clinics, local hospitals, privately funded clinics, and private physicians. Some provide a complete range of services, from information to obstetrics and abortion; most centers refer patients wanting obstetrical, abortion, or sterilization services to hospitals or doctors. In 1981 more than 5 million teenagers were at risk of an unintended pregnancy. Of the 57 percent who received family planning services that year, some 30 percent chose public or private clinics and 21 percent went to private doctors.

Contraceptive services are available if adolescents make an effort to find them; what is needed are ways to strengthen teenagers' motivation to use them. The experience of European countries demonstrates that adolescents can use contraceptives effectively. Unfortunately, in this country several factors hinder contraceptive use, factors that are not a problem in the United Kingdom, France, Sweden, or the Netherlands. They are: a misunderstanding of the benefits and risks of oral contraceptives; a highly visible, fundamental religiousness that is antisexual; racism; and widespread, deep poverty.

Although religiousness and sexual conservatism do not always go hand in hand, in the United States these two characteristics are often closely linked. In the Guttmacher study of teenage pregnancy and child-bearing in 37 nations, the researchers found that in this country a higher proportion of the population attends religious services and believes God is important in their lives. Fundamentalist groups in the United States, which often hold very conservative views on sexual behavior, are both extremely visible and vocal. The nature and intensity of religious feeling in this country tend to introduce more emotion into public discussions about providing reproductive health services to teens than is seen in other countries.

In its prevalence and depth, the poverty that exists in this country is almost unknown in the industrialized countries of Europe. In the United States, one of every five children lives in poverty. Three out of every four black children and one of every four white children experience poverty by age 10; many of them are poor for at least four years. The 37-country study found that in nations with more equitable distribution of family income fewer adolescents become pregnant. Teenagers who have known only poverty and see no hope of escaping it are not likely to feel they are jeopardizing a rosy future by having a child.

With little chance of achieving a sense of satisfaction through work or unstable and sometimes violent family relationships, adolescents living in poverty often see childbearing as a way to achieve something of their own. Consciously or unconsciously, they are apt to view a baby as a source of the love and satisfaction they do not find elsewhere. In some social milieus, having a baby may represent many things to a young man and woman: a way to demonstrate sexual competency and fertility, a sign of adulthood, or a way of relieving the constant stresses of being poor and helpless. When there is no hope of breaking the pattern of generations of poverty, there is little motivation to prevent a pregnancy. Many of these teens may not actively want to have a baby, but they may simply let it "happen" because they see little reason to prevent it.

As noted in Chapter 3, despite the evidence that birth control pills are a safe and effective method for most women, many girls avoid using them because of misinformation and myths regarding their safety and possible side effects. Until their questions about the relationship between oral contraceptives and health and fertility are answered, many young women will continue to avoid using this effective method. What these teenagers don't understand is that the mortality risk associated with adolescent childbirth is greater than the mortality risk associated with the pill.

Besides, oral contraception requires a prescription, a visit to a clinic or private physician for a pelvic examination and a Pap smear, and funds to renew the prescription every month, conditions that while not unsurmountable may be enough to discourage an adolescent from using this effective form of contraception.

In countries where birth control has a high priority, family planning services and birth control methods are subsidized, so the question of cost does not prevent their use. Also, a prescription may not be required for oral contraceptives.

Every form of contraception currently available requires some planning, and researchers find the reason many teenagers give for not using contraception is that they did not expect to have intercourse. Other adolescents may not be ready to admit to themselves that they are sexually active.

Furthermore, each method of birth control currently available in this country has built-in disadvantages. For example, the IUD might have been considered feasible as a contraceptive for adolescents because once inserted it needs little attention. But because the devices have been associated with pelvic inflammatory disease and infertility among women who have more than one sexual partner, manufacturers and epidemiologists now recommend this method be limited to women who have completed their families and are in stable relationships. Long-term methods that might be useful for adolescents are not yet available in this country, although Norplant is expected to become available in 1990. Foams and condoms require no prescription but must be used consistently and carefully to be effective. Diaphragms and cervical caps require instruction in use, have substantial failure rates if not used correctly, and are often viewed as interruptive and messy.

With virtually all methods, younger women tend to experience higher rates of failure; in fact, women under age 22 are about twice as likely as women 30 and older to have an unintended pregnancy while using a contraceptive. The contraceptives available in the United States today are not very appropriate for the teenager whose sexual activity is sporadic and often unanticipated. James Trussell suggests:

> Adolescent pregnancy could be significantly reduced if a safe, relatively inexpensive, non-physician-dependent contraceptive were developed for use

at the end of cycles during which intercourse occurs (thereby eliminating the need to plan ahead).

He adds, however, that such a method would be considered an abortifacient, and abortifacients are not currently eligible for federal research and development support. As mentioned in Chapter 3, RU 486 is available in France and China, but its manufacturers have not yet tried to market it in the United States.

The Use of Abortion

As many studies have shown, almost half the teenagers in this country who become pregnant each year have an abortion. The health risks associated with an early legal abortion are no greater for a teenager than they are for an adult woman. In most instances it is less risky. But the NRC panel found that in states where a parent's consent is required an increasing percentage of adolescent abortions are being delayed, often because the teenager is appealing to the courts for a judicial bypass. Some states do not require parental consent, but the local providers of abortion services do. If the abortion is delayed until the second trimester, the risk to the girl's health increases.

Abortions are performed at 2,680 clinics and hospitals in the United States, with metropolitan areas offering the greatest access to such services. In 1985, 30 percent of U.S. women of reproductive age lived in counties that had no abortion services at all, and 43 percent lived where no major facility performed abortions.

The commitment of many European countries to contraceptive services for teenagers is strongly connected to the desire of those countries to reduce the number of abortions among young women. Originally, conservative physician groups in France and the Netherlands were reluctant to endorse the idea of birth control for adolescents. But they recognized the value of preventive services when it became clear that the alternative would be a rise in teenage abortions. The 1975 law that made abortion legal in Sweden also established the basis of a system for offering contraceptive services to the young, a direct acknowledgment by the government that the need for abortions could be reduced by making effective birth control measures readily available. The attitude of these countries is the opposite of the view held by some groups and influential individuals in the United States that the availability of contraceptive services encourages premarital sex and abortion.

Other Approaches

Some communities and agencies have developed innovative approaches to averting adolescent pregnancy. These include programs that teach assertiveness and decision making, strengthen communication between parents and children, improve school performance, enhance teenagers' views of the future, and increase their job opportunities.

Programs that seek to improve life options for young people are based on the assumption that an adolescent who has realistic goals and a plan for reaching them is less likely to allow early childbearing to interfere with those plans. Most of the current programs are small and experimental, however, and clear-cut results are not yet available.

Some efforts are also under way to raise the consciousness of media executives and help them be more aware of the possible effects on the young of the sexual attitudes portrayed on television. Such media projects also aim to encourage a more responsible approach to the sexual content of programs. More and more professionals and advocacy groups believe that television portrayals of nonmarital sexuality and exploitive and violent sex may contribute significantly to attitudes about sex. Despite the growing concern among professionals and parents, network executives remain reluctant to include in these same programs any mention of contraception or abortion for fear of offending the public. In marked contrast, news programs and talk shows deal boldly with sexual issues, apparently without losing many viewers. Noticeably missing from daily TV fare are programs that portray sexuality in a responsible way as part of stable, long-term relationships. Also missing is national advertising for over-the-counter contraceptives, such as spermicides and condoms.

In the Netherlands and Sweden nonprescription contraceptives are advertised widely in the media; adolescents in those countries have a greater awareness of birth control methods and feel that contraceptives are easily accessible, although there is no hard evidence that such advertising actually has increased contraceptive use among teens. Studies do show that teen pregnancy rates are lower in countries that appear to be less ambivalent about sexuality.

RESEARCH NEEDS

Improving reproductive health in the United States means more research on sexual behavior. Although biomedical research such as that on the relationship between the hypothalamus and puberty may be useful, solutions to the difficult reproductive health problems facing this country are more likely to be found by investigators in the social and behavioral sciences. Many current intervention programs do not have realistic and carefully designed evaluation components built into them. It is important that the outcomes be measurable and that the programs be designed such that outcomes in the study group can be compared with those of a control group similar in every way except for the intervention. The definition of goals and participants and the methods used for making comparisons all need to be precise for research findings to be considered valid.

Such programs would stand a better chance of being replicated successfully and funded adequately if providers were willing to scrutinize their work closely, if researchers were able to evaluate the interventions precisely, and if schools and other sources cooperated by making available the data needed to perform such evaluations.

More research is needed to determine:

• the effects of youth employment projects on teenage sexual behavior and childbearing; in part, that means making the postponement of childbearing a stated goal of such projects.

• how and to what extent special programs to improve school performance are effective in keeping teenagers in school, boosting their achievements, and averting pregnancies.

• the effect on the offspring of living in a family started by an adolescent pregnancy, especially as the children grow up. Such research should control for the relevant background and mediating factors.

• the relationship between early parenting and child development.

• how many adolescents give up their infants for adoption and why they chose this method to resolve their pregnancies. There are currently no systematically collected national statistics on adoption.

• the attitudes of adolescent males toward and knowledge of reproduction and birth control.

• the connection between what young people know and how they behave. Programs may be quite effective in raising the level of knowledge about reproductive behavior without having much impact on that behavior.

• the effect of parental communication and supervision on the sexual activity of adolescents.

CONCLUSION

Although sexual activity among adolescents in the United States is on a par with teenagers in other industrialized countries, this nation has a much higher rates of teenage childbearing and abortion. The reasons for this phenomenon are diverse and not completely defined. However, some are known: the lack of contraceptive use in the United States among many sexually active teenagers; the burgeoning poverty rate and the damaging disadvantages that accompany it; the widespread exploitation of sexuality in the media coupled with a reluctance to show sexual responsibility and the routine use of birth control; and the unwillingness of many segments of U.S. society to discuss sex frankly.

Furthermore, as Guttmacher researcher Elise F. Jones has noted, political and religious leaders in this country appear to be divided about what their goal should be: to discourage sex among adolescents or to concentrate on reducing teenage parenthood by promoting contraceptive use.

Many programs designed to reduce the incidence of teenage parenthood have been undertaken, with unclear results. More projects with well-planned research components are needed to demonstrate clearly what does and does not help adolescents delay sexual activity or avoid pregnancy. Most often, an unintended birth to a teenager limits her education and job opportunities. Until we are able to break the patterns of behavior and economic deprivation with effective intervention programs, teenage parenthood represents a serious threat to the economic vitality of this country.

ACKNOWLEDGMENT

Chapter 4 was based in part on a presentation by Daniel Federman.

REFERENCES

Alan Guttmacher Institute. 1981. *Teenage Pregnancy: The Problem that Hasn't Gone Away*. New York.

Card, J.J., and R.T. Reagan. 1989. Strategies for evaluating adolescent pregnancy programs. Family Planning Perspectives. 21(1):27-32.

Center for Population Options. 1988. *Estimates of Public Cost for Teenage Childbearing in 1987*. Report written by Martha R. Burt. Washington, D.C.

Dash, L. 1989. *When Children Want Children, The Urban Crisis of Teenage Childbearing*. New York: William Morrow and Co.

Forrest, J.D., and R.R. Fordyce. 1988. U.S. women's contraceptive attitudes and practice: how have they changed in the 1980s? Family Planning Perspectives. 20(3):112-118.

Furstenberg, F.F., Jr., J. Brooks-Gunn, and S.P. Morgan. 1987. *Adolescent Mothers in Later Life*. Cambridge, UK: Cambridge University Press.

Henshaw, S.K., J.D. Forrest, and J. Van Vort. 1987. Abortion services in the United States, 1984 and 1985. Family Planning Perspectives. 19(2):63-70.

Jones, E.F. 1986. *Teenage Pregnancy in Industrialized Countries*. New Haven: Yale University Press.

Jones, E.F., J.D. Forrest, N. Goldman, et al. 1985. Teenage pregnancy in developed countries: determinants and policy implications. Family Planning Perspectives. 17(2):53-63.

Kisker, E.E. 1985. Teenagers talk about sex, pregnancy and contraception. Family Planning Perspectives. 17(2):83-89.

National Research Council. 1987. *Risking the Future: Adolescent Sexuality, Pregnancy, and Childbearing*. Washington, D.C.: National Academy Press.

Orr, M.T., and J.D. Forrest. 1985. The availability of reproductive health services from U.S. private physicians. Family Planning Perspectives. 17(2):63-69.

Sege, I. 1989. Poverty's grip on children widens. The Boston Globe. March 12, 1.

Singh, S. 1986. Adolescent pregnancy in the United States: an interstate analysis. Family Planning Perspectives. 18(5):221-226.

Trussell, J. 1988. Teenage pregnancy in the United States. Family Planning Perspectives. 20(6):262-272.

Westoff, C.F. 1988. Unintended pregnancy in America and abroad. Family Planning Perspectives. 20(6):254-261.

Winter, L. 1988. The role of sexual self-concept in the use of contraceptives. Family Planning Perspectives. 20(3):123-127.

Zabin, L.S., M.B. Hirsch, E.A. Smith, R. Streett, and J.B. Hardy. 1986. Evaluation of a pregnancy prevention program for urban teenagers. Family Planning Perspectives. 18(3):119-126.

Zabin, L.S., M.B. Hirsch, R. Streett, M.R. Emerson, M. Smith, J.B. Hardy, and T.M. King. 1988. The Baltimore pregnancy prevention program for urban teenagers: I. How did it work? II. What did it cost? Family Planning Perspective. 20(4):182-192.

5
Prenatal Care
Having Healthy Babies

One of the best measures of a nation's health is its infant mortality rate—the number of babies born alive who die before their first birthday. Because the future of a country depends on the well-being of its children, the health of those children is a major concern.

In highly developed countries the majority of children are healthy. Like much of the industrialized world, during this century the United States made a great deal of progress in reducing the number of deaths among newborns and infants. During the 1980s, however, that progress stagnated; in some U.S. cities infant mortality actually increased.

Although the United States was never a world leader in reducing the mortality rate of its newborns, in 1918 it ranked sixth among 20 selected countries. It wasn't until the 1980s that the United States actually began to lose ground. In 1987, the most recent year for which there are data, the United States ranked nineteenth among industrialized countries in infant mortality, behind such nations as Spain, Singapore, and Hong Kong, where infant mortality rates were 9 per 1,000 births. The lowest newborn death rates are 6 per 1,000 births, found in Japan, Finland, and Sweden.

In 1987 more than 10 out of every 1,000 newborns in this nation died. The death rate for white infants was 8.6 per 1,000 births. The mortality rate for black babies in 1987, however, was close to a staggering 18 per 1,000 newborns, more than twice as high as the rate for white babies. The mortality rate for black newborns in the United States matches the entire national infant mortality rates in Poland, Hungary, Portugal, and Costa Rica, which have the highest infant death rates among 32 nations studied by UNICEF.

The high death rate among newborns in this country is related strongly to the number of infants whose weight at birth is lower than normal for their gestational age or who were born prematurely. Low birthweight is defined as under 2,500 grams (5 lbs. 8 oz.); *very* low birthweight is under 1,500 grams (3 lbs. 5 oz.). Low birthweight is the result of inadequate fetal growth, and the lower the birthweight, the greater the immaturity and risk of death. A number of factors contribute to low birthweight: low socioeconomic status, a low level of education, childbearing very late or very early in the reproductive years, poor nutrition, medical problems, and substance abuse.

By providing necessary medical care and helping pregnant women improve their general health, prenatal care programs play an important role in alleviating risk factors and improving pregnancy outcomes, particularly if the care is adequate and obtained early. In its 1988 study of the health of infants and children, the Office of Technology Assessment (OTA) found that early and comprehensive prenatal care can improve the chances of overcoming low birthweight and infant mortality. Women who do not receive adequate maternity care, on the other hand, double the risk of having a low birthweight baby.

Because low birthweight has such a dominant effect on newborn mortality and on health problems in infants and children, it has become the focus of many professional and public groups. When the National Commission to Prevent Infant Mortality was formed in 1987 to develop a national strategy for reducing infant mortality, its first major report succinctly summarized the current state of infant health in this country:

> What we found is that too many infants are born too small, too many are born too soon, and too many mothers never get decent care and guidance during their pregnancy.

No single reason can explain why the U.S. infant mortality rate stopped declining in the 1980s. Infant mortality is rooted in a broad, saddening array of factors such as poverty, absent fathers, physical and emotional abuse, poor housing, lack of parenting role models, and, increasingly, drug abuse.

One factor worth noting is the growing number of births of extremely tiny infants of approximately 500 grams (about 1 lb.) who are resuscitated but subsequently die. Some observers believe that the changes in managing and reporting the births of these extremely immature infants are partly responsible for leveling the infant mortality rate.

Furthermore, many professionals are concerned that the deepening poverty in this country and the steady decline in public funding for health services are having a negative impact on maternal health and infant mortality. While 48 states offer some prenatal care programs for poor women, restrictive eligibility requirements and a scarcity of clinics mean that such programs reach only a small percentage of the women who need them. In addition, during the recession of the early 1980s, many breadwinners lost their jobs and with them the employer-paid health insurance that often covered prenatal care. The Congressional Research Service reports that virtually all the increase in the number of uninsured Americans since 1980 is the result of declining employer-based coverage of dependents.

Many factors lead to the increase in infant mortality seen in this country, but this chapter concentrates on the important interactions between prenatal care, birthweight, and infant survival. It reviews the current status of health care services for women and babies in the United States, particularly the services available for pregnant women, since such care influences the health of the next generation. The chapter also surveys the many barriers that make prenatal care difficult to obtain for the very women who need it most.

MATERNAL AND INFANT HEALTH—THE PICTURE TODAY

Key measures of the health of an industrialized society are its rate of infant mortality, its percentage of low birthweight newborns, and what proportion of its pregnant women receive prenatal care. From the mid-1960s to the 1980s, the United States made considerable improvement in these areas. During the 1980s, however, progress toward reducing infant mortality stalled.

Among blacks, in 1985 and 1986 the national decline in infant deaths became so small it was statistically insignificant. For every state that recorded improvement in its mortality rate for black infants, there was a state in which the rate climbed. On a state-by-state basis, black infant mortality rates ranged from 12.7 to 24 per 1,000 births. The average was 18 deaths per 1,000 births, which is significantly higher than the national average of 10.4 percent for all races. The death rate for white infants ranged from 7.7 to 11.3 per 1,000 births.

Year-to-year fluctuations in the mortality rates for both black babies and white babies are to be expected, but observers at the OTA believe that the slowing of the decline in the infant mortality rate in this decade cannot be dismissed as a random variation in the trend.

The U.S. newborn death rate is related in large part to the high percentage of low birthweight infants. The United States ranks twelfth in the number of infants born with low and very low birthweights. Low birthweight is an important determinant of infant health and mortality. Most low birthweight babies are immature, which means they are born before they reach their normal growth and development in the uterus. As a result, they are more likely to die during infancy or to become children who require more medical care and hospitalization than the average child. Analysts at the Children's Defense Fund find that immaturity contributes to two-thirds of the deaths of babies in their first month of life. The OTA reports that in 1980 low birthweight infants represented less than 7 percent of all newborns in the United States but accounted for 60 percent of all babies who died in infancy.

LOW BIRTHWEIGHT AND INFANT MORTALITY

Birthweight came to be viewed as an measure of fetal growth early in this century; a low birthweight was seen as an indicator of inadequate intrauterine growth or prematurity and the baby was not expected to live. Forty years ago the World Health Organization (WHO) adopted 2,500 grams (5 lbs. 8 oz.) as the weight below which newborns were considered to be of low birthweight. Although a low birthweight was often associated with an abbreviated gestation, in 1960 the WHO noted that this was not always true. An infant weighing less than 2,500 grams was not always premature but, instead, could be small for its gestational age.

Before 1950 most infant deaths occurred after the first month of life, generally as a result of environmental factors such as infections and poor nutrition. As the incidence of such deaths fell by mid-century, there was a shift in the timing of infant deaths. After the 1950s the majority of infant deaths occurred during the neonatal period, the four weeks immediately after birth. The causes of those deaths were rooted in the pregnancy and birth process and included birth injuries, asphyxia, congenital defects, and low birthweight.

The latter is a significant factor. In 1950 only 7.5 percent of newborns weighed 2,500 grams or less, yet two-thirds of the infant deaths that year occurred in among such low birthweight babies. Beginning in the

1960s the relationship between birthweight and infant mortality has been documented frequently in several countries and hospitals. The studies reveal that, compared with infants weighing a more normal 3,000 to 3,500 grams (6 lbs. 5 oz.) and up, babies weighing less than 2,500 grams are almost 40 times more likely to die in the weeks after their birth. The likelihood of death increases as birthweight decreases. If small babies survive the neonatal period, they continue to have a higher risk of death during their first year, accounting for 20 percent of infant deaths during that period.

Major advances in improving infant mortality have been achieved through saving the lives of premature infants, not in reducing the prevalence of low birthweight. In the late 1960s sophisticated monitoring and treatment methods were developed for premature infants whose undeveloped lungs did not function properly. In the 1970s neonatal intensive care units (NICUs) became part of most large hospitals. In the 1980s improvements in respiratory therapy and mechanical ventilation began to make it possible to save the lives of newborns with very low birthweights of less than 1,500 grams (3 lbs. 5 oz.).

The widespread use of NICUs is associated with a small percentage of children growing up with neurodevelopmental handicaps. Some have physical impairments that are the result of the technology itself. How serious these problems are as the child grows older and begins school and how they are affected by socioeconomic and other factors is not yet fully understood.

Babies born in hospitals with NICUs have a better survival rate than those born in hospitals without them. By reducing the death rate of very small newborns, NICUs have been the principal means for the decline in U.S. infant mortality rates in recent years. In reviewing the 1986 data, observers at the Children's Defense Fund conclude:

> Any decline in the national neonatal mortality rate in 1986 presumably was not achieved because more infants were born healthy. Rather, more fragile infants survived the newborn period with the aid of expensive hospital technology.

In contrast, the enhancement of infant birthweight, which would improve the outcome for so many newborns, has been so slight that it has had little impact on mortality figures.

Some observers suggest that neonatal mortality rates ceased to drop because the reporting of births of extremely small newborns, those weighing less than 500 grams (about 1 lb.), has increased at many hospitals.

From 1981 to 1984 the number of reported births of these tiny infants rose more than those in any other category of birthweight in the United States. Almost all of these infants died during the newborn period. In earlier years such babies usually did not survive the birth process and were listed not as births but simply as fetal deaths. Today in many places they are counted as live births and, subsequently, as infant deaths. Some analysts believe one factor in the current slowdown of the infant mortality decline may be this difference in managing and reporting extremely immature births, rather than a real deterioration in the health of pregnant women.

POVERTY AND INFANT MORTALITY

Others concerned with the rate of infant mortality in this country believe that an important factor in infant mortality rates is the progressive "dis-insurance" of the working poor, the increase in the proportion of women and infants living in poverty, and the shrinking in real dollars of subsidized health services for pregnant women and children.

Poverty increases the chances of producing a low birthweight baby. The incidence of premature birth and inadequate fetal growth is greater among poor women. The causes are not clear; however, Paul H. Wise, of Harvard, and Alan Meyers, of Boston University, note there is evidence that prematurity and inadequate growth are related to elevated risk and reduced access to medical care:

> Poor nutrition, small stature, increased stress, and obstetric complications can all affect birth weight and are more common among poor women. A risk often overlooked is the state of a woman's health prior to conception. In this context, the effect of poverty on birth outcome may represent in part a legacy of inferior health status of poor women both before and during their childbearing years.

Decreased spending on publicly funded health care in this country during the 1980s has paralleled the increase of poverty among women and children. In its 1988 book, *Healthy Children: Investing in the Future*, the OTA reports that from 1978 to 1984 the percentage of infants residing in poor families rose from 18 to 24 percent. At the same time, Medicaid expenditures in constant dollars per child recipient declined by 13 percent and federal funding for three important sources of primary health care for poor women and children—maternal and child health services, community health centers, and migrant health centers—declined in constant dollars by 32 percent.

Sara Rosenbaum of the Children's Defense Fund and her co-investigators found in 1986 that in 15 states hospitals denied admission to women about to deliver babies. In another 13 states hospitals were refusing to admit women who were not in "active" labor. "Patient dumping" was recorded in 6 other states. The researchers also found that one or more hospitals in 23 states required a cash deposit if a woman wanted to preregister for delivery. A woman who could not pay a deposit would not be admitted for delivery unless she was in advanced labor and was considered an emergency case.

The OTA found that putting health care out of the reach of increasing numbers of poor women and children would have had only a "modest effect" on the overall infant mortality rate by the mid-1980s. However, the report also pointed out:

> Yet, for a particular infant, being born to a mother in poverty with limited access to prenatal and infant care substantially raises the risk of dying in the first year. Thus, cutting back on funding for health care services at the same time that infant poverty rates in this country were increasing raised the risks of infant mortality for these babies.

THE EFFECTS OF LOW BIRTHWEIGHT

Helping low birthweight newborns to survive is often only part of the medical care they will require. The Institute of Medicine (IOM) Committee to Study the Prevention of Low Birthweight, convened in 1982, found that many of these babies are at increased risk for a number of health problems, which in turn engender financial and family stresses. In its 1985 report, *Preventing Low Birthweight*, the committee notes "this increased risk has implications for health services, and possibly for educational services and family function as well."

Health Problems

Neurodevelopmental Handicaps

The most obvious side effect of low birthweight is the substantial prevalence in these youngsters, as they grow, of such neurodevelopmental handicaps as cerebral palsy, seizure disorders, and other neurologically based deficits. Low birthweight infants are three times as likely as normal-weight babies to have neurological problems, and the risk increases with every decrease in weight level.

Congenital Anomalies

Because defects can cause premature birth, immature infants are twice as likely as newborns of normal weight to have a serious inborn defect; in very immature babies these anomalies occur three times as often. They range from having extra fingers or toes, strabismus (a condition in which the muscles that control the eye are weak, affecting eye alignment and vision), to serious brain or heart defects.

Respiratory Tract Problems

The lungs of low birthweight babies often are immature, and the infants may have respiratory distress syndrome or hyaline membrane disease. As they grow up, such children may experience repeated lower respiratory tract infections and abnormal lung functioning. The persistence of these problems is particularly common among children who as newborns required prolonged ventilator support.

Side Effects of Technology

The technology used today to diagnose and treat low birthweight newborns can have deleterious effects on the baby. Best known is the effect of oxygen administration on the eyes of immature infants: It may cause retrolental fibroplasia, severely damaging eyesight and sometimes causing blindness.

The increased incidence of problems experienced by low birthweight babies means a greater use of health care services. In its report on these infants, the IOM committee said:

> The length of hospital stay in the neonatal period for infants who survive to the first year of life averages 3.5 days for normal birthweight infants, but is much longer for smaller infants: 7 days for those between 2,001 and 2,500 grams at birth; 24 days for those between 1,501 grams and 2,000 grams; 57 days for those less than 1,500 grams; and 89 days for those less than 1,000 grams.

The committee found that in addition to the lengthy hospital stays many of these babies require when they are born, a substantial proportion of very immature newborns are rehospitalized during their first year and require more physician visits.

Family Stresses

Not surprisingly, the birth of an immature infant who requires intensive hospital care and may have chronic, sometimes disabling physical problems can produce tremendous stress on the family. The bonding between mother and baby often is disrupted, and a great deal of anxiety is produced by the infant's critical condition. These factors can also have a negative effect on later parenting behavior and on the interaction between the parents and the child.

Financial Stresses

The cost of the intensive medical care needed by immature infants frequently is enormous. Even families with insurance still must pay as much as 20 percent of hospital charges. Families without insurance often must pay as much as one-third of the total hospital bill. According to studies by the Alan Guttmacher Institute, the average bill for the delivery and care of a healthy baby is about $4,300, or one-fifth of the income of a typical young couple.

If the birth is complicated, the bill can easily be higher. The OTA found that in Maryland in 1986 the extra cost for hospital care for a low birthweight infant was $5,236. (That year the average hospital cost per admission in Maryland was within one-half percent of the national average.) A study at the University of Pennsylvania found that if an infant was discharged earlier and received follow-up nursing care at home, the cost of its hospitalization could be reduced by 25 percent, lowering the hospital charge for the infant's medical care to an average of $3,763. The average 1986 hospital charge for the care of a normal-weight newborn was $658.

Low birthweight babies have higher rates of respiratory, gastrointestinal, and infectious illnesses than do infants born at normal weights. Compared to normal-weight newborns, twice as many low birthweight babies are rehospitalized at least once during their first year. The extra cost of rehospitalization is conservatively estimated by the OTA at about $800 per low birthweight child. This does not take into account doctors' fees or the high rates of hospitalization of very sick premature infants who did not survive infancy.

A large proportion of low birthweight infants are born to families living in poverty and to teenage mothers who do not qualify for Medicaid under individual state criteria. In many of these cases the cost of care for a low birthweight child is carried by the hospital and passed on to the public. In addition, many working families have no health insurance or have insurance that provides only limited coverage. As a result, the cost of caring for low birthweight babies is borne by the public.

PREVENTING LOW BIRTHWEIGHT: THE ROLE OF PRENATAL CARE

Studies demonstrate that infant mortality and low birthweight can be alleviated if the pregnant mother receives sustained, quality medical care beginning early in her pregnancy, so that incipient problems can be detected and corrected before they affect the fetus. Newborns whose mothers had no prenatal care are almost five times more likely to die than babies born to mothers who had early prenatal care. Good comprehensive care includes screening for potential problems; education and counseling about the connection between nutrition, life-style, and pregnancy outcome; and medical treatment as needed.

Almost all studies of prenatal care have some methodological short-comings; despite this, a review of more than 55 studies by the OTA revealed that the weight of evidence "supports the contention that two key birth outcomes—low birthweight and neonatal mortality—can be improved with earlier and more comprehensive prenatal care, especially in high risk groups such as adolescents and poor women."

COST-EFFECTIVENESS OF PRENATAL CARE

Although the value of prenatal care is unquestioned, what is not yet clearly understood is exactly which preventive measures are effective and when during a normal pregnancy they should be applied. Also unresolved are questions regarding which components of prenatal care are most healthful and cost-effective and how best to reach the women who most need such care.

The OTA performed a cost-effectiveness analysis to determine how health care system costs would be affected if all pregnant poor women were enrolled in Medicaid, a policy made possible by the Omnibus Budget Reconciliation Act of 1987. "Poor" in this instance refers to women with incomes below 100 percent of the federal poverty level. The OTA estimates that offering such Medicaid eligibility would bring an additional 18.5 percent of poor women into prenatal care during their first trimester at a national cost of $4 million annually. The OTA also

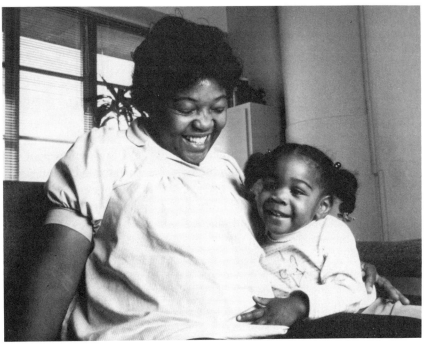

To assure the best possible outcome for a mother and her baby, medical care plus nutritional, educational, and other support services are vital. Credit: National Institute of Child Health and Human Development

estimates that, for every immature birth prevented by better prenatal care, the U.S. health care system saves between $14,000 and $30,000 in expenses for newborn hospitalizations and long-term health services. For the savings to outweigh the costs, between 133 and 286 low birthweight births would have to be averted nationally among the newly eligible Medicaid users of early prenatal care.

Current evidence suggests that it is indeed feasible to reduce the number of low birthweight births considerably well beyond the breakeven point. Several reasonably well-designed studies on the relationship between early prenatal care and birthweight have demonstrated effects that were at least twice as great as the effects needed for the Medicaid expansion to pay for itself. The OTA notes that early prenatal care also can prevent an unknown number of newborn deaths.

A study by Theodore Joyce and his colleagues at the National Bureau of Economic Research compared the cost-effectiveness of various

health inputs and government programs in reducing race-specific neonatal mortality or death during the first four weeks of life. They found
that early prenatal care was the most cost-effective strategy for reducing
newborn mortality among both black and whites. Their analysis also
revealed that blacks benefited more per dollar of resource use. Although
neonatal intensive care was the most effective method of reducing infant
mortality, it was one of the least cost-effective.

For the IOM study on the prevention of low birthweight, analysts
calculated how fiscal outlays for the medical care for low birthweight
infants might be reduced if expenditures for prenatal care for high-risk
pregnant women were increased. They estimated that each $1 spent
on prenatal care might save over $3 in medical care for such infants,
if increasing the amount of prenatal care decreased the rate of low
birthweight from the current 11.5 percent to the 9 percent level, the
Surgeon General's 1990 goal for high-risk women.

The IOM committee observed that averting low birthweight births via
comprehensive prenatal care will also reduce the risk of such disabling
conditions as cerebral palsy and mental retardation, which frequently
require long-term public assistance.

WHO ISN'T GETTING ENOUGH PRENATAL CARE?

Many women in the United States do not receive sufficient care:
those who are still in their teens; who are black, Hispanic, or American
Indian; who are unmarried; who are recent immigrants; who have less
than a high school education; and who live in poverty. Each year at least
1.3 million women receive insufficient prenatal care, and many of them
are the women who most need it.

Sufficient care is best defined as the amount needed to produce both a
healthy baby and a healthy mother. The amount of care received in prenatal programs varies in the number of visits and therapeutic interventions.
The American College of Obstetricians and Gynecologists (ACOG) and
the American Academy of Pediatrics (AAP) have issued guidelines, but
professionals disagree about the amount and content of prenatal care for
normal pregnancies, about what constitutes a high-risk pregnancy, and
about methods for handling high-risk pregnancies.

The ACOG and AAP guidelines call for maternity care visits to begin
as early as possible during the first 3 months of pregnancy, continuing
every 4 weeks until the 28th week, every 2 to 3 weeks until the 36th
week, and then every week until delivery—a total of 13 to 15 visits. Such

guidelines focus primarily on the number of visits rather than on their content. The OTA found that in the United States in 1984, 20 percent of white babies and 39 percent of black babies were born to mothers who had no prenatal visits during their first trimester. A substantial proportion did not even see a doctor until they were 7 months pregnant.

When the rate of adequate care rather than the trimester in which care was first obtained was reviewed, the prenatal care picture darkened. A 1985 study by Dana Hughes and others for the Children's Defense Fund found that only 68.2 percent of all women obtained adequate care, 23.9 percent received an intermediate level of care, and 7.9 percent had inadequate care. The definition of adequacy was based on a modified version of the Kessner Index, which cross-tabulates the timing of the first doctor's visit with the total number of visits made and the length of the pregnancy.

Teenagers

The percentage of babies born to mothers receiving late or no prenatal care varies significantly by age. Of all age groups, pregnant adolescents are the least likely to receive early prenatal care. This delay in receiving care is linked to the much-noted high risk of teenagers having low birthweight infants. In 1986 there were 472,081 births to women under the age of 20; 1 in 5 babies born to girls under age 15 and 1 in 8 born to mothers between ages 15 and 19 were low birthweight newborns. Almost 14 percent of all the low birthweight infants born in the United States in 1986 were born to adolescents under age 15, and 9.3 percent were born to adolescents aged 15 to 19.

Unmarried Women

Childbearing by unmarried women is on the increase in the United States. The greatest rate of this increase currently is among white women, although a black infant is still four times as likely as a white infant to be born to an unmarried woman. In 1986 the National Center for Health Statistics revealed that 23.4 percent of all births in this country were to unmarried women, a 6 percent increase over 1985. Unmarried women are much more likely to be poor, especially if they are adolescent mothers. As the Children's Defense Fund analysts note:

> The proportion of births to unmarried women of all ages continues to increase, placing families at greater risk of poverty. In 1987 one in every

two children living in female-headed households was poor. Among very young children living in households headed by single mothers younger than twenty-two, 88.8 percent were poor in 1987.

Blacks, Hispanics, and Native Americans

Black women are far less likely than white women to receive early prenatal care; they are twice as likely to receive no care or to obtain it late. Black infants are much more likely to die of causes that are usually considered preventable through comprehensive prenatal care.

Similarly, except for those of Cuban background, Hispanic women are much less likely than white women to begin prenatal care during the first trimester and three times as likely to receive either no care or late care. Cuban women, however, often are privately insured and are more accustomed than white women to begin prenatal care early.

In 1985 there were approximately 41,000 births to American Indian women and 112,000 to Asian or Pacific Islander women. Hawaiian women and other Asian subgroups, such as Cambodian, Vietnamese, and Korean, received late or no care at a rate somewhere between black and white women. Native American women were the most likely of all ethnic groups to receive insufficient care.

Immigrant women are also at greater risk of receiving little or no care during their pregnancies. Differences in local health care systems, language, and ethnic attitudes toward such care may keep them from obtaining prenatal services.

The Poorly Educated

The IOM Committee to Study Outreach for Prenatal Care, which began its work in 1986, found that education was an important factor in receiving prenatal care. The timing of the first prenatal visit correlated highly with education levels. In 1985, 88 percent of mothers who had some college education began care during their first trimester, while only 58 percent of women who had less than a high school education sought care early. The effect of education may be modified by ethnicity and other factors.

Women with Many Children

The more children a mother has, the less likely she is to obtain prenatal care. Fourteen percent of women pregnant with their fifth child received late or no care, compared with close to 5 percent of mothers having their first or second child.

Women Living in Poverty

Poverty is one of the most important factors consistently associated with insufficient prenatal care. A review of the data from the 1980 National Natality Survey shows that women whose incomes were at or below 150 percent of the federal poverty level were three times more likely to receive no prenatal care or late care than women whose incomes were equal to or above 250 percent of the poverty level. An analysis of data from the 1982 National Survey of Family Growth found that only one-half of women living below the federal poverty level obtained maternity care in their first trimester of pregnancy. The 1985 Massachusetts prenatal care survey revealed similar findings: Only 38 percent of women with yearly incomes of less than $10,000 obtained adequate prenatal care, while adequate care was received by 64 percent of women whose incomes fell between $10,000 and $20,000. When family income reached the $40,000 to $50,000 level, the percentage went up to 88 percent.

Growth in real family income has been slowing since 1973, and between 1979 and 1986 the median adjusted income for the bottom two-fifths of all families fell 2 percent. Families with children have made no gains in real income despite a 16 percent increase in the number of working mothers. Economic burdens are particularly heavy for those with a family head under age 25. Between 1970 and 1986 the real median income of those families dropped by 43 percent. Because the minimum wage in terms of real dollars has declined 33 percent since 1981, a person with two children who works full time at the minimum wage will earn $2,500 less than the poverty level.

The Uninsured

Between 1978 and 1985 the number of Americans without insurance multiplied from 28 million to more than 35 million. Nearly one-fourth are young adults aged 18 to 24, including millions of young women in their peak childbearing years. Three-fourths of Americans who were uninsured in 1984 were workers and their dependents. Public health specialist Lorraine V. Klerman emphasizes that employment is no guarantee of either general health benefits or pregnancy benefits. Studies find that many women are employed in companies that do not offer health insurance. Unemployed women may not be covered by the insurance of their spouses or fathers.

Companies that employ fewer than 15 or that self-fund their insurance plans may not offer maternity benefits. Retail and service organizations, such as fast-food restaurants, where many women find employment, often do not offer comprehensive health insurance. Part-time workers seldom receive any medical coverage. Furthermore, the rapidly increasing costs of health benefits are leading many employers to drop part or all of their health insurance plans. Young couples, who have the preponderance of babies, often begin their work careers in jobs that pay poorly and provide inadequate health insurance coverage. Furthermore, young wage earners seldom have enough savings to cover gaps in their insurance.

The Alan Guttmacher Institute found that in 1985 a total of 14.6 million women of childbearing age had no insurance coverage for maternity care. Of this number, 9.5 million women had no health insurance of any kind. Those most likely to be uninsured are teenagers and poor women who either are unemployed or are working at low-paying jobs. Their lack of insurance poses a serious problem, because they are most at risk for adverse (and expensive) pregnancy outcomes if they do not get early and comprehensive care.

Dr. Klerman also pointed out that women who do have maternity coverage may still not get adequate maternal care because of limits in benefits or because their coverage requires substantial cost sharing—strategies that are becoming increasingly common as the cost of health insurance rises. Medicaid covers only a small proportion of the poor.

A University of California, San Francisco, study found that in eight counties in California the number of newborns without health insurance rose by 45 percent between 1982 and 1986. The lack of health insurance was associated with an elevated and still-rising risk of adverse outcomes for the infants. The number of newborns requiring hospital stays longer than 6 days rose from 9,975 in 1984 to 14,411 in 1986. The researchers believe that the escalating risk of detrimental outcomes in uninsured newborns is "explained most plausibly by diminished access to care, together with other factors related to lower socio-economic status."

OBSTACLES TO PRENATAL CARE

Inability to Pay

Studies suggest that one of the most important reasons women do not obtain adequate prenatal care is their inability to pay for it. As previously noted, many women do not have enough money to pay clinic or private physician fees, and many either have no insurance or their insurance policies do not cover maternity care. Although the 1978 Pregnancy Discrimination Act requires employer-based health insurance to include maternity benefits, the law applies only to the employee and spouse. As a result, 35 percent of typical family policies do not cover dependents such as teenage daughters for maternity care.

Only 25 percent of employer-based policies provide coverage for a teenager and her baby. This major gap in insurance coverage poses a serious problem because these young women are at especially high risk for adverse pregnancy outcomes and need early prenatal care.

Since its 1965 enactment, Medicaid has become the largest single source of health care financing for the poor, making medical services more accessible to more low-income individuals and families. Data from the National Center for Health Statistics reveal substantial increases between 1969 and 1980 in the number of women enrolling in Medicaid in order to receive early prenatal care. After 1981, however, the number remained static. After a survey of 51 Title V Maternal and Child Health agency officials in 1986, Sara Rosenbaum and her fellow researchers observed:

> As private insurance coverage of the poor has ebbed, the growing deficiencies of the Medicaid program, the nation's largest public financing system for low income families, have grown more glaring.

The women who have enrolled in Medicaid have not obtained care as early or as often as women who have private insurance. There are numerous reasons: (1) In some states, Medicaid enrollment can be so time-consuming that many mothers are well into their pregnancies by the time they are eligible for care. (2) Medicaid enrollees often rely on clinics for care, and in some communities such clinics are so overcrowded that appointments must be scheduled for many weeks away. (3) Many private physicians who provide maternity care are unwilling to accept Medicaid or nonpaying patients, and others have reduced the number of such cases they will see. (4) Pregnant women on Medicaid often are, by definition, at the bottom rung of the economic ladder and are characterized by many other demographic factors associated with not seeking prenatal care, such as being under age 20, unmarried, and in fair or poor health.

In an effort to provide health insurance for more poor pregnant women, Congress passed new laws between 1984 and 1988 that made it possible for states to expand their Medicaid eligibility standards. The effect of one of the laws was to sever the connection between Medicaid and AFDC. The 1986 Omnibus Budget Reconciliation Act (OBRA) allowed states for the first time to offer Medicaid to pregnant women who had incomes up to 100 percent of the federal poverty level regardless of whether they were eligible for AFDC under the rules of an individual state. Forty-five states adopted this expansion. The 1988 Medicare Catastrophic Coverage Act required that all states extend their Medicaid coverage to this level by mid-1990.

Furthermore, the 1987 OBRA gives states the option of providing maternity care benefits to all pregnant women and infants whose family incomes are at or below 185 percent of the federal poverty level. The Children's Defense Fund in 1989 estimated that if all states exercise this option Medicaid eventually will be available to cover health care costs for nearly one of every two births in the United States.

Because some restrictive eligibility standards remain, however, a large proportion of near-poor pregnant women and infants still are ineligible for Medicaid assistance.

A Shortage of Clinics

It has been well documented that in some areas public health clinics, community health centers, and outpatient departments that could provide maternity care are in short supply. At the same time, the number of women who are uninsured and unable to pay for their maternity care is growing because the proportion of women who work part time or in low-paying jobs with limited or no health benefits also is growing. For these women publicly financed clinics are the only available resource. The shortage of clinics has led to long waiting times before a pregnant woman can be seen by clinic staff for an initial prenatal visit. Waiting periods are so long at some clinics that it is not possible to see every pregnant patient during her first trimester. Expanding clinic hours may not be possible if funds are not available to pay for additional staff time.

The IOM prenatal care study committee found numerous examples of overcapacity and a shortage of services:

• In 1985 a survey of its 42 public health clinics by the Los Angeles County Department of Public Health found that waits for initial prenatal visits ranged from 2 to 14 weeks.

• In Charleston, West Virginia, from 1982 to 1986 at least one clinic closed admissions periodically every year, sometimes for as long as 2 months, because its limited staff could not keep up with the high volume of patients.

• During a 3-month period in 1986, public clinics in San Diego County were forced to turn away 1,245 women seeking prenatal care because the clinics were filled to capacity. Orange County, California, clinics could not give appointments to 2,000 women in 1985. Officials in these counties estimated that at least half the women who could not be cared for at the county health centers were unable to find care anywhere else.

• A 1982 survey of private nonprofit New York City hospitals found waiting times that ranged up to 4 months for a first prenatal appointment.

Although community health clinics offering maternity health services have never been in oversupply, in recent years federal budget cuts coupled with a recession have forced local health departments to reduce their staffs at a time when the need for their services increased markedly. Some reported reducing or eliminating maternity or nutrition services, or both.

Physician Inaccessibility

The need for publicly supported prenatal care services has been exacerbated by a decrease in the availability of obstetricians and family practitioners who provide maternity care. Although the United States has no shortage of physicians overall, some areas do not have enough doctors and others have none at all. For example, Mississippi reported in 1983 that 51 of its 82 counties had no resident obstetrician. Eleven of 58 counties in California did not have an obstetrician and 9 of those counties had no public prenatal care clinic. Although the number of practicing obstetricians has been increasing, many areas still have few or none.

The presence of an adequate number of practitioners, however, does not make maternity care more accessible to poor and uninsured pregnant women, unless the physicians are willing to accept Medicaid or to reduce their fees for women who have no maternity coverage at all. Among primary care physicians, obstetricians have been the least likely to accept Medicaid patients, according to an early 1980s study of physician access.

In a 1984 survey of primary care physicians, 36 percent of obstetricians said they did not provide care to Medicaid patients. By comparison, 25 percent of general practitioners, 23 percent of pediatricians, and 20 percent of internal medicine practitioners did not accept Medicaid patients. Physicians give many reasons for refusing to accept Medicaid patients: extensive paperwork, slow claims processing, long-delayed and uncertain payments, and reimbursement rates that represent only a fraction of the physician's actual costs or usual fee. This latter claim is borne out in a comparison of Medicaid versus the usual obstetric fees, which include prenatal care. Usual charges in 1986 averaged $830 for a vaginal delivery; the average Medicaid reimbursement was $554. Medicaid reimbursement rates have risen in recent years, yet they remain substantially lower than customary physician charges. In addition, the IOM prenatal care study committee reported:

> The problem of low Medicaid reimbursement is exacerbated by the high proportion of Medicaid women who are high-risk patients. Because of multiple health and social problems, these women often need more frequent and comprehensive maternity care than more affluent women, and such extra care can be time-consuming and expensive to provide.

Indeed, the case could be made, the committee says, that because many pregnant women enrolled in Medicaid are at high risk, reimbursement for their care should be greater than the average obstetrical fee.

Restrictions on Nurse-Midwives

In both rural and urban areas, certified nurse-midwives and nurse practitioners have been especially effective and experienced in managing the care of high-risk pregnant women. Obstetric customs and, in many states, legal restrictions have limited the number and the scope of practice of nurse practitioners and nurse-midwives. Although in many European countries they provide the majority of maternity services, in the United States only some 2,600 nurse-midwives are actively practicing.

THE COST OF MALPRACTICE INSURANCE

Malpractice insurance premiums for practitioners who provide obstetrical services doubled between 1982 and 1985. The reasons are many and include changes in medical technology, changing standards of practice, and an increase in large awards and in the size of lawyer contingency fees.

Premium costs and increasing anxiety about the risk of a malpractice suit have driven many providers to discontinue their obstetrical services or to cut back the number of their obstetric patients. When the ACOG surveyed its members in 1983 and 1987, it found that, because of malpractice concerns, the proportion who reduced the number of high-risk patients they saw had increased from 18 percent to 27 percent. These physicians also had decreased the number of deliveries they performed, and a substantial number said they had stopped practicing obstetrics entirely.

A similar member survey by the American Academy of Family Physicians in 1986 revealed that 23 percent had stopped providing obstetric services because of malpractice concerns.

The malpractice situation has a particularly negative effect on public clinics, which are having a difficult time obtaining liability insurance and finding physicians willing to practice obstetrics. Chronically underfunded inner-city health centers often are forced to eliminate obstetric services because they cannot afford the insurance. As Sara Rosenbaum and Dana Hughes of the Children's Defense Fund point out:

> Even though both Community Health Centers and nurse midwives have very low malpractice claims profiles compared to other providers of obstetrical care, their rates have risen dramatically. . . . At one center in Florida, malpractice coverage for prenatal care services is $4,000 annually per staff member. Coverage for delivery, however, would add $25,000 in costs per staff person.

Dr. Klerman advises that physicians may use the fear of malpractice suits as a reason for reducing or eliminating their Medicaid or uninsured caseload, due to an unsubstantiated belief that these women are more likely to sue. The recently published IOM study of medical professional liability and the delivery of obstetrical care found that this perception by physicians is not supported by the data available.

The committee notes that people with low incomes generally have less access to the legal system. In addition, medical malpractice actions are brought by attorneys on a contingency fee basis. Because awards usually are based on lost earnings, among other things, it would appear that attorneys have less financial incentive to serve poor plaintiffs. A Government Accounting Office study of malpractice claims found that the average expected payout for a Medicaid plaintiff was $52,000; the average for a privately insured plaintiff was $250,000.

Most studies regarding the relation of income to medical malpractice suits do not bear out doctors' perceptions that they are at greater risk of being sued by poor or Medicaid patients.

The Programs

Lack of Coordination Among Programs

Five principal federal programs supply prenatal care and related services to low-income women: Medicaid; Maternal and Child Health Services Block grants; the Special Supplemental Food Program for Women, Infants, and Children; community health centers; and migrant and rural health centers. Each has a different function and, if they could work together, they would furnish pregnant women with many of the maternity services they need.

Unfortunately, the programs often are not well coordinated at the community level; their connections to other public services and to private physicians range from weak to nonexistent. The IOM prenatal study committee found that coordination between programs can be difficult because each is independently organized and has its own administration, rules, and constraints. A woman may be eligible for Medicaid coverage and for prenatal care services from a local health department clinic, but enrolling in both may require meeting different eligibility standards, applying at different sites, completing different applications, and furnishing different documentation.

Pregnancy testing services are another example of poor coordination among programs. Although testing services may provide the telephone numbers of prenatal clinics, many services do not have close ties to prenatal care clinics. The lack of a direct relationship does not help women whose pregnancy tests are positive to make an appointment for the important first-trimester evaluation. Close ties to prenatal care clinics would expedite appointments, making it easier for clients to start maternity care.

Medicaid Application Procedures

Medicaid is the major source of payment for prenatal services obtained by pregnant poor women, yet rates of enrollment among women eligible for the program vary as much as 11 to 84 percent from state to state, and many eligible women do not enroll. The reasons are many. Medicaid programs rarely publicize their benefits or explain how to enroll, and their brochures seldom note that pregnancy may be grounds for eligibility. Although a few states have streamlined their enrollment procedures, in many they often are excessively complicated. Application forms can run from 4 to 40 pages, and a typical form may include 80 to 100 questions. Completing an application often requires two or three trips to the Medicaid office and long waiting times, and eligibility can be denied on the basis of a single missing document, such as a utility bill. In addition, eligibility must be redetermined periodically during pregnancy; changes in household composition or expenditures can stop Medicaid coverage in the middle of a pregnancy, unless the state has adopted the continuous eligibility option. The long waiting periods between making an application and receiving a Medicaid card make it difficult to receive prenatal care during the first trimester. Even physicians and clinics who accept Medicaid as payment may insist that the enrollment process be completed and the patient have her card in hand before they schedule an appointment.

As the IOM committee observed,

> The difficult application process, the complexity of the program and the great variations in the program across states create the impression of a system designed to discourage rather than encourage entry into prenatal care.

Although the committee noted that Congress and the states have taken steps recently to broaden Medicaid eligibility, it also observed that the program remains limited in its ability to draw low-income women into prenatal care promptly and with a minimum of bureaucratic harassment.

Other Barriers

The traditional obstacles to receiving early and regular care continue to hinder women from receiving necessary services. Long-standing barriers include the following.

Transportation

These impediments to care include the need to travel long distances to reach a clinic, the high cost of transportation, and no means of transportation at all. In some cities poor neighborhoods have limited public transportation services, and rural areas often have no bus or rail services. The IOM committee pointed out that the lack of a car and the transportation problems that result have become a mark of poverty and can form insurmountable barriers to obtaining health services.

Child Care

If a woman already has children, her use of prenatal health services is affected by the availability of child care. If she can not find or afford a babysitter, she may have to bring her children with her. If there are long waits at the clinic and child care is not provided, the burden of taking the children may outweigh any perceived benefits of the visit.

Clinic Hours

The problems of accessibility created by the need to travel long distances, inadequate transportation, and lack of child care are exacerbated by limited clinic hours. Most clinics are open only on weekdays from 8 or 9 a.m. to 5 p.m., making it difficult for women who work or go to school to schedule appointments. Women in low-paying jobs lose wages for time not worked or risk disapproval for taking time off. When some District of Columbia clinics began offering prenatal appointments during the evening and weekends, the number of patients seeking care at those clinics increased markedly.

Long Waiting Times

Long waits are common in publicly financed health centers, particularly in those using the block appointment system. In that system women are told to come either at 8 or 9 a.m. or at 1 p.m., and then they are seen on a first-come, first-served basis. For most patients this means a wait of 2 to 3 hours, an experience patients describe as frustrating and humiliating. It can also be costly in terms of time lost from work or in child care expenses. A study of low-income prenatal care patients in New York City found that the women viewed long waiting times as a sign of the staff's disregard for the value of their time; they said it was especially insulting to wait several hours and then have only a few minutes with a physician.

Staff Attitudes

The use of prenatal care can also be influenced by the way clinic staff treat patients. Seeing a different doctor each time, receiving hurried or impersonal care, and dealing with rude or indifferent appointment clerks or receptionists discourage patients from continuing prenatal care. Socioeconomic differences between staff and patients may add to an already negative atmosphere, and language differences compound the problem. Even something as simple as not having enough chairs for waiting patients conveys the message that the patients are not wanted.

Hiding the Clinic

Few clinics let prospective patients know the clinic location or how they can make appointments. Studies report that 5 to 18 percent of women who received little or no prenatal care before the birth of their child did not know where to find such services. The IOM committee found that few telephone directories have a listing for "prenatal care" or a similar phrase.

Cultural and Personal Barriers

Personal attitudes and the cultural characteristics of the pregnant woman can also impede adequate prenatal care. The IOM panel found that the use of prenatal care is affected by the woman's attitude toward her pregnancy and prenatal care, whether she views such care as useful, and by her cultural values and beliefs, her life-style, and certain psychological characteristics.

Attitudes

Whether a woman makes an effort to find prenatal care appears to depend on how she regards her pregnancy. If it is unplanned and she views it negatively, she is more likely to delay care and to make infrequent clinic or physician visits. Accordingly, most observers feel that a reduction in unplanned pregnancies would lessen the incidence of late care.

Not all women feel that prenatal care is important. Some believe that pregnancy is a normal function and that medical care is needed only when a pregnant women is unwell.

Failure to recognize the signs of pregnancy also is a factor in delaying care. Studies demonstrate that between 16 and 33 percent of the women who did not receive sufficient care did not know for some time that they were pregnant. This is particularly true of first-time pregnant women, especially those still in their teens. "Not knowing I'm pregnant" also is a form of denial, a marker of an unintended and usually unwanted pregnancy.

Fears can be substantial barriers. They can include fear of medical personnel or procedures, fear of the reaction of others to the pregnancy, fear that one's status as an illegal alien may be discovered, and fear of pressures to change life-style habits such as substance abuse, smoking, or eating disorders. For some women the stress and pressures of their lives may prevent them from obtaining adequate prenatal care. Anxiety about lack of money, housing difficulties, difficulties with the baby's father, lack of emotional support, and other problems can interfere with finding care.

Denial also interferes with the use of prenatal care. Although this can be seen in women of any age, it is most prevalent among teenagers. As noted in Chapter 4, some adolescents simply do not want to believe that they can get pregnant. The denial continues into pregnancy. Frank F. Furstenberg's survey of teenage mothers in Baltimore found that half the adolescents did not tell their mothers about their pregnancy until several months had elapsed.

These psychological problems are difficult to correct, particularly through public policy procedures, Dr. Klerman observes. But she believes that increased funding for Medicaid and for public prenatal clinics, changes in private insurance regulations so more women are covered for maternity care, and aggressive outreach and educational campaigns will help appreciably and are within the scope of national and state legislative concerns. She adds that, "Attention should be paid to these items, rather than blaming the victim for neglect of needed care."

Homelessness

Not surprisingly, women who are homeless and living in shelters have difficulty obtaining prenatal care. Forty percent of pregnant women living in hotels for the homeless in New York City during 1982 and 1984 received no care at all.

Substance Abuse

Pregnant women who are aware that their life-styles risk their health and the health of their babies may also be afraid to seek care because they expect pressure to change such habits as heavy smoking, eating disorders, or the abuse of drugs or alcohol. Substance abusers, especially, may avoid seeking prenatal care because of the disorganization and stress in their lives. They also fear that their drug use will be discovered, they might be arrested, and their other children might be taken into custody.

Several recent studies show that a significant number of women in the childbearing years of 18 to 35 frequently use cocaine and other drugs. Substantial percentages of women who obtain prenatal care late or not at all abuse drugs, particularly heroin and cocaine. The number of babies who test positive for a variety of illegal drugs is increasing steadily in the United States, particularly in large cities. The babies of drug-using mothers often have multiple problems that may require intensive care and long hospital stays: low or very low birthweight, drug addiction, neurodevelopmental disorders, and congenital defects.

A study of 75 cocaine-using mothers and their infants by Dr. Ira Chasnoff, of Northwestern University Medical School, found that many women who use cocaine become pregnant without realizing it and continue to use the drug. Even if they give up cocaine after the first trimester, these women remain at high risk for miscarriage. If they continue to use cocaine throughout their pregnancy, they increase their risk of having a preterm delivery and a low birthweight infant or of having a full-term baby who is smaller than normal.

A study of 1,226 infants and mothers at Boston City Hospital by Barry Zuckerman and other researchers from Boston University had similar findings. All the women were drawn from the prenatal clinics held by the hospital. Approximately half the women used marijuana or cocaine; in all other demographic characteristics, including use of cigarettes and alcohol, the women's backgrounds were similar. Drug use was determined by urinanalysis, self-reporting, or both. The majority of mothers in this study were low-income women and most were single.

In all measures of newborn growth, the infants whose mothers used marijuana or cocaine were significantly smaller than the babies born to nonusers. In addition, babies born to cocaine-abusing mothers were at greater risk of being premature. With one exception, congenital malformations were not significantly more frequent among babies born to mothers who used these two drugs. Among the babies of cocaine users, however, the proportion of one major or three minor congenital problems was considerably larger (14 percent versus 8 percent) than among the infants of nonusers.

Dr. Zuckerman and his colleagues point out that many of the women who used drugs also exhibited a life-style associated with depressed fetal growth. They used alcohol and cigarettes, and the pregnant cocaine users also were found to have a greater incidence of sexually transmitted diseases. Cocaine users weighed less before pregnancy and gained less during its course. In the presence of these multiple risk factors, the researchers note, the use of cocaine or marijuana further impairs fetal growth. Although pregnancy may serve as an impetus for a woman to stop using alcohol or cigarettes, drug users appear to find it much more difficult to abstain during pregnancy.

RESEARCH NEEDS

Although many agencies and programs help provide health care to pregnant women and young children, increasing numbers of pregnant women do not receive maternity care until the third trimester or obtain no care at all. Health care professionals have suggested several approaches for drawing into care those low-income women who are at elevated risk for poor pregnancy outcomes. Some advocate scrapping current national programs and instituting a new comprehensive one; others recommend changing current services so they can reach more women and provide care in a coordinated, user-friendly way. More research is needed on these issues:

• A basic understanding of the mechanisms that underlie inadequate intrauterine growth and the premature onset of labor is necessary to develop preventive measures.
• The programs that are most successful in bringing women into prenatal care early and in keeping them there should be identified.
• When financial and access barriers are reduced, what can be done to bring into care those women who have psychological problems or educational deficits that prevent them from seeking prenatal care?
• Do regular home visits by health care personnel help increase a pregnant woman's compliance with medical recommendations? What is the minimum number of visits that are useful?
• What programs are successful in helping pregnant women change the life-styles that endanger the health of the fetus?
• What services can be offered to drug-addicted women and how and where should such services be made available in order to keep these women in care both for their pregnancy and to treat their addiction?
• Teenagers and other young unmarried women need to be made more aware of the importance of prenatal care; identifying the most influential and cost-effective components of educational programs would be useful before large-scale efforts are designed.

CONCLUSION

Since the beginning of this century, the infant mortality rate in the United States has steadily declined. That decline slowed during the 1980s, showing almost no progress from 1984 to 1986. Several factors are implicated in this leveling off of infant deaths: a deepening of poverty in the United States; a more careful reporting of extremely low birthweight infants who die almost immediately, which in the past would have been reported as fetal deaths or would have gone unreported altogether; a continuation of the large proportion of births to teenagers and unmarried women, who often have low birthweight babies; and an increase in the percentage of women receiving prenatal care late or not at all.

The effect of these factors has been exacerbated by an increase in the number of women, particularly young women, who are not covered by maternity insurance, by the difficulty and the delays that pregnant women experience when they try to enroll in Medicaid, by a decline in the number of physicians accepting low-paying Medicaid patients, and by a lack of coordination among clinics. In general, the picture is one of more women being at risk for having babies who are preterm or whose fetal growth has been retarded, while at the same time services to improve the health of such mothers and their infants are reduced and fragmented.

ACKNOWLEDGMENT

Chapter 5 was based in part on a presentation by Lorraine V. Klerman.

REFERENCES

Alan Guttmacher Institute. 1987. *Blessed Events and the Bottom Line: Financing Maternity Care in the United States.* New York: The Alan Guttmacher Institute.

Braveman, P., G. Oliva, M.G. Miller, R. Reiter, and S. Egerter. 1989. Adverse outcomes and lack of health insurance among newborns in an eight-county area of California, 1982-1986. New England Journal of Medicine. 321:508-513.

Brooten, E., S. Kumar, L. Brown, et al. 1986. A randomized clinical trial of early hospital discharge and home follow-up of very low birthweight infants. New England Journal of Medicine. 315:934-939.

Chasnoff, I., D.R. Griffith, et al. 1989. Temporal patterns of cocaine use in pregnancy. Journal of the American Medical Association. 261:1741-1744.

French, H.W. 1989. Tiny miracles become huge public health problem. N.Y. Times, February 19.

Gold, R.B., A.M. Kenney, and S. Singh. 1987. Paying for maternity care in the United States. Family Planning Perspectives. 19(5):190-206.

Hughes, D., K. Johnson, S. Rosenbaum, and J. Liu. 1989. *The Health of America's Children: Maternal and Child Health Data Book*. Washington, D.C.: Children's Defense Fund.

Institute of Medicine, Committee to Study Medical Professional Liability and the Delivery of Obstetrical Care. 1989. *Medical Professional Liability and the Delivery of Obstetrical Care: Volume I*. Washington, D.C.: National Academy Press.

Institute of Medicine, Committee to Study Outreach for Prenatal Care. 1988. *Prenatal Care: Reaching Mothers, Reaching Infants*. Edited by Sarah S. Brown. Washington, D.C.: National Academy Press.

Institute of Medicine, Committee to Study the Prevention of Low Birthweight. 1985. *Preventing Low Birthweight*. Washington, D.C.: National Academy Press.

Joyce, T., H. Corman, and M. Grossman. 1988. A cost-effectiveness analysis of strategies to reduce infant mortality. Medical Care. 26:348-360.

Kleinman, J.C., and S.S. Kessel. 1987. Racial differences in low birth weight. New England Journal of Medicine. 317:749-753.

McCormick, M.C. 1989. Long-term follow-up of infants discharged from neonatal intensive care units. Journal of the American Medical Association. 261:1767-1772.

Moore, T.R., W. Origel, T.C. Key, and R. Resnik. 1986. The perinatal and economic impact of prenatal care in a low-socioeconomic population. American Journal of Obstetrics and Gynecology. 154:29-33.

Murray, J.L., and M. Bernfield. 1988. The differential effect of prenatal care on the incidence of low birth weight among blacks and whites in a prepaid health care plan. New England Journal of Medicine. 319:1385-1391.

National Center for Health Statistics. 1989. *Advanced Report of Final Health Statistics, 1987*. Monthly Vital Statistics Report. Vol. 38, No. 5 Supplement. September 26.

National Commission to Prevent Infant Mortality. 1988. *Death Before Life: The Tragedy of Infant Mortality*. Washington, D.C.: National Commission to Prevent Infant Mortality.

Rosenbaum, S., D.C. Hughes, and K. Johnson. 1988. Maternal and child health services for medically indigent children and pregnant women. Medical Care. 26:315-332.

Schur, C., A.B. Bernstein, and M.L. Berk. 1987. The importance of distinguishing Hispanic subpopulations in the use of medical care. Medical Care. 25:627-641.

U.S. Congress, Office of Technology Assessment. 1988. *Healthy Children: Investing in the Future*. OTA-H-345. Washington, D.C.: U.S. Government Printing Office.

U.S. Congress. 1989. House Select Committee on Children, Youth, and Families. *Children and Families: Key Trends in the 1980s*. 100th Congress, Second Session, 1989. Washington, D.C.: U.S. Government Printing Office.

Wise, P.H., and A. Meyers. 1988. Poverty and child health. Pediatric Clinics of North America. 35(6):1169-1186.

Zuckerman, B., et al. 1989. Effects of maternal marijuana and cocaine use on fetal growth. New England Journal of Medicine. 320:762-768.

6

Progress in Research

The absence, since 1980, of the Ethics Advisory Board has, in effect, put a moratorium on federal funding for research on many aspects of reproduction. As a result, basic research studies in this field are few and many questions remain unanswered. As noted in earlier chapters, the lack of basic information has slowed the development of contraceptives and the improvement of infertility treatments. We still do not understand important aspects of the human reproduction system, the process of fertilization, the type of gene activity that occurs as a fertilized egg divides, and the best way to assay embryonic cells for the range of chromosomal and genetic defects that cause disease. In this chapter are described three examples of research areas that hold much promise: the role of the brain in reproduction, new methods of diagnosing genetic diseases, and research on embryo health.

ROLE OF THE BRAIN IN REPRODUCTION

Research makes it clear that the brain governs most aspects of reproductive functioning. The hypothalamus appears to be the command center that governs the action of several hormone-driven loops that are part of the operation of the reproduction system. The reproduction processes of both sexes in all vertebrates, down to the fishes, are the consequence of a cascade of neuroendocrine events initiated in the hypothalamus.

The discovery that ovulation depends on the regularity of the hypothalamic stimulation of the pituitary gland has had immediate application to patient treatment. Working with monkeys, Dr. Ernst Knobil, of the University of Texas, found that the ovulatory cycle is controlled by the regularity with which the hypothalamus stimulates the pituitary gland to release gonadotropins into the circulatory system. If the pattern is altered in any way, ovulation stops within a week or two. If the regular pulses of hormone are re-established, normal ovulation begins again. Today ovulation is being restored to an increasing number of women by means of the timed delivery of a key hormone.

The hypothalamus is affected by nerve and hormonal inputs from other parts of the body. When these inputs are in the normal range, the hypothalamus responds by producing pulses of gonadotropin-releasing hormone (GnRH), which stimulate the pituitary gland into releasing luteinizing hormone (LH) and follicle-stimulating hormone (FSH), the gonadotropin hormones. The gonadotropins, in turn, act on either the testes in the male, regulating sperm production, or the ovaries in the female, regulating the ovulatory cycle.

The hypothalamus controls the body's ability to reproduce. In all animals the timing of pregnancy is tailored by biological evolution. In some mammals, including humans, the hypothalamus integrates information about body weight, stress, exercise, and overall health. If these inputs indicate that a female is well nourished and able to sustain the stress of pregnancy and lactation, the hypothalamus secretes gonadotropin-releasing hormone in regular pulses, and regular ovulatory and menstrual cycles begin. Many modern women experience amenorrhea, the absence of menstruation, as a result of physical and psychological stresses. A study in Sweden found that 3 to 4 percent of women suffer amenorrhea for three months or longer during the course of a year in response to various stresses. Amenorrhea also occurs when the female body becomes too lean through starvation, rigorous exercise, or eating disorders.

Through its control of important hormones, the hypothalamus is the ultimate controller of the onset of egg and sperm development. In the male and in the female, this part of the reproductive system is complete and functional at birth but soon afterward becomes dormant. Then, some months before puberty, a still unknown mechanism gradually activates the reproduction-controlling function of the hypothalamus. When the pulses of gonadotropin-releasing hormone reach the pituitary at the proper frequency, the pituitary responds by producing gonadotropins. Menstrual cycles begin in girls, and in boys sperm production gets under way.

Dr. Knobil noted that a variety of factors can negatively influence the pulses of GnRH. Opiates like morphine can slow or stop the pulses entirely. Stress, habitual strenuous exercise, and malnutrition, including anorexia nervosa, also affect it, halting menstruation and ovulation.

Research by Drs. Stephanie Jofe and William F. Crowley, of the Harvard Medical School, found that in 1,600 women (physicians, post-doctoral researchers, and medical students) the incidence of amenorrhea was approximately 3 percent, the same as that for women in other occupations. The shutdown of hypothalamic function in most of these women could be explained by a poor state of nutrition, a recent illness, a program of rigorous exercise, or grief. The ordinary stresses and strains of life did not appear to be a major factor in causing hypothalamic amenorrhea, Dr. Crowley notes.

According to Dr. Crowley's studies, the hypothalamus produces bursts of GnRH in a pattern that varies during the ovulatory cycle. In women whose cycles are normal, the rate of these pulsations speeds up before ovulation and then slows down dramatically until menstruation, when it largely ceases. To restore normal ovulation to women with hypothalamus-based amenorrhea, Dr. Crowley and his team treated them with round-the-clock doses of GnRH. The hormone was given intravenously in 4- or 5-microgram pulses via a beeper-size pump worn by the patient. The pump was programmed to deliver GnRH in pulses that ranged in frequency from one every 60 or 90 minutes or once every 4 to 6 hours, a pattern that mimics the natural timing of the hypothalamus. By copying the normal rhythm, Dr. Crowley achieved a 93 to 95 percent success rate in restoring normal ovulation to more than 100 women with amenorrhea. At present, this treatment is available from medical centers only for primary amenorrhea; approval for treatment of other forms of the disorder is expected from the Food and Drug Administration by late 1990.

Not all scientists agree about the importance of keying the changes in the pulsing rate exactly to those that occur naturally, but they do agree that the critical feature in the reproductive hormone network is the delivery of GnRH into the blood circulation in small regular bursts. Some clinicians are able to restore ovulation by administering GnRH every 60 or 90 minutes; the results improve, according to Dr. Crowley, when the treatment most closely follows the innate rhythm of the hypothalamus.

Males have the same network of neurons in the hypothalamus that integrate nerve and hormone signals from the rest of the body and produce GnRH in a regular pulsating pattern, stimulating the pituitary to release the LH and FSH gonadotropins. In males these gonadotropins drive the production of the male sex hormones and, in turn, of sperm. If the hypothalamus is influenced to stop secreting pulses of GnRH entirely or if secretion becomes irregular, sperm development is stopped or reduced. Tony M. Plant, of the University of Pittsburgh, is looking for an association among a particular pulsatile pattern of gonadotropin secretion, a change in the important ratio between LH and FSH, and reduced sperm count. What remains to be known is the exact morphologic and physiologic nature of this neuronal system: what starts the firing, what controls its duration, and what stops it as abruptly as it began.

DIAGNOSING GENETIC DISEASES

The increasing ability of medical scientists today to diagnose genetic disorders is making it possible for more couples who may carry the genes for an inherited disease to give birth to healthy babies. Before medical scientists were able to detect the presence of such genes, couples who risked passing on an inherited disease often chose not to have children. Today, thanks to tests that reveal whether a person is or is not a carrier for a genetic disorder or whether or not a fetus has the disease, couples can make informed decisions about having a child.

Genetic diagnosis includes identifying adults who might pass along inherited disorders to their children, screening newborn babies for congenital diseases that would be disabling without an intervention, and detecting genetic disorders in the fetus. Tests include examining chromosomes for structural abnormalities and identifying genetic diseases in infants by detecting the presence or absence of certain chemicals in the body. An example of the latter is the use of a blood test to identify babies born with phenylketonuria (PKU). Such children cannot metabolize the amino acid phenylalanine, which accumulates in the blood and prevents the brain from developing normally. A special diet averts mental retardation.

More recently, genetic diseases are being identified more directly with analyses of DNA, that can reveal the absence of a gene or the presence of a faulty gene. In PKU, for instance, the defective gene is located on chromosome 12. These new techniques are making it increasingly possible to diagnose genetic diseases prenatally.

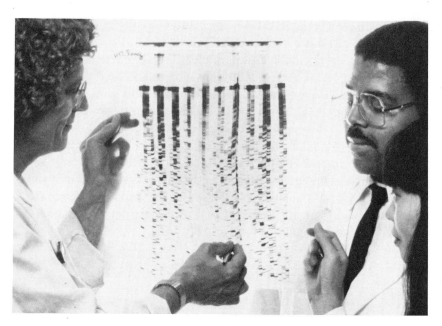

Researchers study the results of a DNA analyzing technique to find a defective gene sequence. Credit: National Institute of Child Health and Human Development

On the horizon are techniques for examining embryos before they are artificially implanted for chromosomal abnormalities and defective genes. If procedures to diagnose genetic and chromosomal defects in early-stage embryos are developed successfully, couples at risk for passing on a genetic disease could be offered in vitro fertilization as a way to have a healthy child. If such technology becomes available, an embryo's chromosomal makeup could be analyzed in advance and only embryos with normal chromosomes and genes would be transferred to the uterus.

HOW GENETIC DISEASES OCCUR

In the cells of every living thing are genes that, working together, direct the structure and function of every type of cell. Genes are the code, or set of instructions, by which an individual cell replicates and produces certain enzymes and other chemicals vital to the development and function of each individual living thing, whether it is a corn plant or a human being.

Although cells may have specialized functions—intestinal cells make mucus and heart cells contract rhythmically—their basic components are similar. Each cell has an operating center, or nucleus, and in that nucleus are the chemical compounds we know as chromosomes, the genetic material we inherit from our parents that determines how the cell will function. The most important component of a chromosome is DNA, deoxyribonucleic acid. DNA is a long, twisted, double chain of chemical compounds called nucleotides. Genes are sequences of nucleotides. Some genes are formed of relatively short sequences; other genes are very long. The DNA of each chromosome is composed of thousands of genes.

Human cells contain 46 chromosomes that look like short bits of fine thread; during cell division the chromosomes form into 23 pairs. Half of each pair contains genes from the mother; the other half comprises genes inherited from the father. As a cell divides, the chromosomal DNA replicates, so the new cell will contain the same genetic instructions as the original.

Sometimes as a cell divides, one of the gene sequences is deleted or altered. Scientists suspect that every human being inherits about 20 altered, or mutated, genes that may have the capacity to harm. A single altered or missing gene may not cause a noticeable problem, because the child has a normally functioning gene on the companion chromosome inherited from his other parent. But if the mutation is transmitted to a child and that child also receives the same mutated gene from the other parent, severe and sometimes fatal diseases can result. This rarely occurs in a heterogeneous population, but in small closed societies where there is a lot of intermarriage, the odds are substantially increased and a gene mutation can eventually become quite prevalent. Today a number of inherited diseases are associated with certain ethnic groups.

Thalassemia, for instance, is a hereditary, often fatal, blood disease common to people of Mediterranean descent, chiefly Italian and Greek. It includes different forms of anemia. In severe cases, children appear healthy at birth but soon become listless, pale, and prone to infections. They grow slowly. The only treatment is frequent blood transfusions, which eventually lead to iron accumulations in the organs and early heart failure. A person who carries the gene for thalassemia will have one normal gene and one thalassemia gene. He or she generally will have no symptoms or only mild symptoms of the disease. But if both parents are thalassemia carriers, there is a two in four chance that their child will inherit one normal and one thalassemia gene and be a carrier for the disorder. Moreover, there is a one in four chance the child will inherit either both normal genes or both thalassemia genes. If the latter occurs, the child will have a severe form of thalassemia.

DIAGNOSIS BY ANALYZING DNA

In recent years, as scientists have learned how to locate defective genes among the thousands that compose DNA, a highly sophisticated field of diagnostic testing has come into existence. One of the many hereditary biochemical disorders of metabolism is Lesch-Nyhan syndrome, in which the body does not produce an essential enzyme. This syndrome is characterized by severe mental retardation, stiff limbs, and self-mutilation. Although the boys (Lesch-Nyhan is a sex-linked disease) born with this disease may live for many years, they often must be restrained to prevent them from severely hurting themselves. Today cells taken from the amniotic fluid during pregnancy can be examined for the gene mutation responsible for this disease, allowing parents to decide whether they want to carry the pregnancy to term.

Most genetic tests are performed on an individual basis for persons who know or suspect they are at risk for passing along a disease. Or such tests may be part of a hospital-based genetic counseling service. Like genetic tests, prenatal tests are done on an individual basis when parents fear their offspring might be born with a serious disability or fatal illness. For some diseases, however, technology makes broad screening programs of adults and newborns possible.

Adult Screening

If the genetic test for a disorder is fast, accurate, reliable, and inexpensive and if the population at risk can be defined, wide-scale screening for carriers is feasible. Tay-Sachs disease is an example in which relatively inexpensive screening has markedly reduced its incidence. The disease is found chiefly among Jews of European ancestry; screening programs for Tay-Sachs have detected more than 15,000 carriers and have identified some 800 couples at risk for having a baby with the disease. Prenatal tests give such at-risk couples the option of carrying to term only normal children. In 1970 between 50 and 100 babies with this fatal disease were born; today fewer than 10 are born each year.

Similar screening for carriers has been attempted for sickle cell anemia and thalassemia. In some community-based screening programs, a blood sample for testing was taken when a couple applied for a marriage license. The programs were never successful, largely because of inadequate educational efforts, lack of confidentiality, and concern about stigmatization.

Screening Newborns

Approximately 12 percent of inherited metabolic diseases can be treated successfully. In order to find the infants who could benefit from such therapies before long-lasting damage can occur, screening programs for these diseases are mandatory in many countries and in most parts of the United States.

The tests require small samples of blood and urine; a few drops of blood taken from the baby's heel shortly after birth are all that is necessary to test for PKU and more than 10 other disorders. If PKU is identified in an infant immediately after birth, for example, the baby can be put on a special low-protein diet right away to prevent phenylalanine accumulation.

Urine is collected by putting a piece of filter paper in the baby's diaper three or four weeks after birth and sending the paper to a laboratory. Among the diseases identified this way are homocystinuria (high levels of homocystine in the blood), galactosemia (an accumulation of galactose), and maple syrup urine disease, a derangement of amino acid metabolism that gives a maple syrup odor to the baby's urine. Like PKU, these metabolic disorders cause mental retardation and other serious problems; if treated promptly, they can be completely or partially controlled by diets designed to circumvent the child's inability to metabolize the particular chemical.

Because the tests are simple and relatively inexpensive, it is feasible to do them for every newborn. The cost of the test is outweighed by the savings in medical care that would be required if the disease were not arrested at a very early stage.

Prenatal Testing Techniques

Many serious birth defects occur without any known cause, and no prenatal test is available to detect them early in a pregnancy. For some of the most common, however, such as Down syndrome and certain neural tube defects, prenatal tests do exist. The majority of these prenatal tests depend on biochemical assays to detect the evidence of a genetic disease. For several genetic diseases, however, new techniques that analyze fetal DNA to find the markers closely linked to the diseases are now available at some medical centers. If an abnormality is detected, the couple can decide if they want to abort the fetus. Today the following prenatal tests are available:

Amniocentesis is a technique in which a small amount of the amniotic fluid surrounding the fetus is withdrawn via a needle. The test is used primarily to examine the chromosomes for evidence of Down syndrome and other disorders caused by errors in the chromosome structure. The amniotic fluid also can reveal the presence of by-products of disease, such as abnormal enzymes or abnormal protein molecules. One drawback of conventional amniocentesis is that detection is limited to those diseases that leave evidence in the amniotic fluid itself or in the cells that can be found in the amniotic fluid. Another drawback is that the fluid cannot be withdrawn until after the 14th week of pregnancy, when the womb can be easily felt. Also, the fetal cells must grow in the laboratory for 1 to 3 weeks in order to have enough to analyze. The results of an amniocentesis generally are not known for several weeks, at which point an abortion can be physically and emotionally difficult. About 1 in 200 women miscarry after amniocentesis.

Fetal blood testing involves drawing blood from the umbilical cord via a needle guided by ultrasound through the mother's abdomen. Fetal blood can be tested for infectious diseases, for evidence of abnormal metabolism, and for defective genes that account for blood diseases such as thalassemia, sickle cell disease, hemophilia, and chronic granulomatous disease, a disorder that affects males, making them very vulnerable to bacterial infections. Umbilical blood cannot be sampled until the blood vessel has grown large enough, which is around the 16th week of pregnancy. The risk of pregnancy loss for this test is not yet fully known; at some medical centers with much experience with fetal blood sampling, the risk appears to be about 1 percent; otherwise it may vary from center to center.

Chorionic villus sampling (CVS) makes it possible to test fetal cells between the 9th and 11th weeks, much earlier than with an amniocentesis or fetal blood test. The chorionic villus is part of the developing placenta and in most cases possesses the same genetic information as the fetus. A snippet of this tissue is taken either via a catheter that is inserted through the birth canal into the uterus or with a needle through the mother's abdomen. Because the procedure collects more live cells than does amniocentesis, the cells do not have to be grown in a culture, so CVS requires less laboratory time. Parents receive results much earlier in the pregnancy, when an abortion is physically less draining. CVS does have a disadvantage, however: It does not always carry the same genetic information as the fetus during early development.

A multicenter study that compared CVS with amniocentesis found that the rates of fetal loss and failure for CVS vary widely from hospital to hospital. The investigators suggest the technique be performed only at medical centers that commit adequate resources to perform the procedure and that perform a substantial number of them. The study found that in experienced hands the spontaneous abortion rate for chorionic villus sampling is 0.8 percent higher than for amniocentesis.

Ultrasound technology has vastly improved since its debut in the 1970s, and, in the hands of an experienced physician with a good knowledge of fetal anatomy, it is a useful diagnostic tool. The clear, real-time images of today's ultrasound can reveal a number of skeletal disorders, defects in the central nervous system such as anencephaly (an extremely small head indicating defective brain development) and hydrocephalus (an excessive accumulation of fluid in the brain). Urinary tract obstructions and kidney defects can also be detected with ultrasound.

Maternal serum alpha-fetoprotein screening (MSAFP) is used to measure the levels of alpha-fetoprotein (AFP) in the blood of pregnant women. AFP is produced by the fetal liver; a small amount passes into the maternal blood circulation, with the concentration gradually increasing until late in the pregnancy. A *high* level of AFP early in a pregnancy can indicate that a woman is carrying a fetus with spina bifida, in which the spinal column has not closed, and other related defects of the central nervous system. Very *low* levels of AFP are associated with a somewhat increased chance of Down syndrome, but the extent of the risk depends on the mother's age. At present, the MSAFP screen is performed between the 16th and 18th weeks; research is under way to make it possible to do this important assay between the 9th and 12th weeks.

Alpha-fetoprotein is a screening mechanism, not a precise diagnostic test. The finding of an unusually high or low level of AFP primarily indicates a need for additional evaluation. The test must be done by a laboratory experienced in MSAFP testing and the results correlated with the age and race of the mother and the week of the pregnancy. Experience with AFP screening programs demonstrates that of 1,000 pregnant women tested, 50 may have high levels of AFP in their blood. Of those 50 women, further testing is likely to reveal that two have fetuses with structural defects of some kind. About one-half of the women with high AFP levels may be at higher risk for complications later in their pregnancies and should be closely monitored by their physician or clinic.

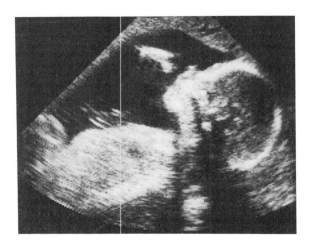

This sonogram of a 21-week-old fetus was one of a series made to evaluate potential kidney problems before birth. There is a history of kidney disease in this family. A healthy baby boy was born in July 1989.

New Techniques for Diagnosing Genetic Diseases

Conventional prenatal tests are useful only if the affected cells are accessible to a sampling method and if scientists know what biochemical changes or products to look for. Today, in addition to detecting diseases by means of biochemical assays of the disease by-products, scientists are using recombinant DNA technology to analyze fetal cells for certain defective genes that lead to disease. This rapidly developing technology is the most important advance in the field of prenatal diagnosis over the past decade.

Recombinant DNA techniques are particularly valuable in detecting inherited diseases that cannot be discovered by biochemical tests. For example, PKU cannot be diagnosed before birth by a biochemical assay because the abnormal enzyme associated with the disease can be found only in liver cells. Fetal liver cells are not collected by amniocentesis, fetal blood sampling, or chorionic villus sampling. However, because all cells carry all the genes of a particular individual, PKU—and a continually growing number of other genetic diseases—can be diagnosed prenatally by using DNA analytical techniques to examine fetal skin or blood cells. Today it is possible to identify prenatally the genes that account for cystic fibrosis, sickle cell anemia, and thalassemia. Sickle cell anemia is a blood disorder that affects large populations, chiefly of African origin; cystic fibrosis causes chronic lung infection that often leads to an early death.

DNA analytic techniques show promise for distinguishing even elusive genetic alterations. For example, although the gene mutation that leads to Lesch-Nyhan syndrome is highly variable in its mutations, this technology enables researchers to locate it. Dr. C. Thomas Caskey, a molecular geneticist at the Baylor College of Medicine, has studied 50 Lesch-Nyhan patients thus far and no two families have had the same gene mutation.

The techniques are becoming more automated and simplified, making it possible to scan a region where a gene sequence may occur in hours, rather than days. One method can find a Lesch-Nyhan gene deletion in approximately 4 hours; the previous test required 7 days. A second method uses direct sequencing of amplified DNA to detect a single base pair mutation in 2 days, replacing a more complicated process that requires several months.

Gene mutations associated with human disorders are identified by comparing normal DNA patterns with the chromosome known to have the mutated gene. Often before the gene itself is pinpointed, chromosomal landmarks, or markers, are used to locate its approximate position. Markers are variations in DNA that are easier to identify and close enough to the gene to be inherited with it. Much medical research is devoted to finding markers linked to specific inherited disorders. When such a marker is identified, it can be used to distinguish healthy chromosomes from those carrying the defective gene. Finding the defective genes themselves remains important, however, because only in a given family may markers be reliable indicators of the presence of a gene. Moreover, identifying the faulty gene is the necessary first step toward developing a treatment to replace it or to alleviate its disease-causing activity.

DNA analytical methods that detect such markers are being improved and broadened. Dr. Caskey notes that new technologies being used to distinguish the genetic mutations for Lesch-Nyhan syndrome also make it possible to detect with great efficiency the many deletions that can occur in the extensive Duchenne muscular dystrophy gene. Duchenne muscular dystrophy is characterized by progressive muscle weakness, usually ending in death before age 20. The test is done prenatally, using tissue from the chorionic villi, and results are available to the parents in 2 or 3 days.

138

SCIENCE AND BABIES

RESEARCH ON EMBRYO HEALTH

Although physicians and researchers have made remarkable advances in their ability to diagnose genetic diseases in human fetuses, only in the last few years have human eggs, sperm, and preimplantation embryos been studied for abnormal genes and chromosomes. Such studies in this and other countries have been limited by ethical concerns regarding the sources of embryos used for research.

Flawed Chromosomes and Pregnancy

Spontaneous abortion, especially early in a pregnancy, is a common event. Based on studies made between 1938 and 1953 by Arthur Hertig and John Rock at Harvard, scientists have calculated that one-half to two-thirds of all conceptions do not result in a live birth. Geneticist Aubrey Milunsky, of Boston University, observes that as many as one-third of all recognized pregnancies end in spontaneous abortion and another 22 percent are lost before or at the time of the first menstrual period after conception. In his book, *Choices, Not Chances,* Dr. Milunsky also notes:

> Among the most common causes of miscarriage are disorders of the chromosomes of the developing embryo or fetus. Recent estimates imply that 1 in 10 sperm or eggs carries a chromosome abnormality.

In 1978 a method was developed for analyzing the chromosomal complement in human sperm. Sperm from healthy men were found to have abnormalities at an average frequency of 8 to 9 percent. More recently, investigators in Italy, England, Sweden, France, and Canada found that substantial percentages of both eggs and embryos exhibit chromosomal defects. At his IVF clinic in Cambridge, England, Dr. Robert G. Edwards and his co-workers found that 30 percent of the embryos they examined microscopically before implantation had defective chromosomes. When Michelle Plachot and her colleagues in Paris analyzed both eggs and embryos, they found that 30 percent of the eggs and 26.1 percent of preimplantation embryos were chromosomally abnormal. In a Swedish study of infertile women undergoing ovulatory stimulation, a team led by Dr. Hakan Wramsby found that nearly 50 percent of the eggs recovered were abnormal.

In almost every instance the eggs and embryos being studied were from infertile women and had been donated for study by infertility clinics because they were no longer needed. Because they came from infertile, often older women, the eggs and embryos may have had a higher than average rate of abnormalities. In turn, Dr. Plachot believes the high rate of chromosome defects in those embryos may account for the high level of implantation failures and the later fetal losses experienced by women receiving IVF treatment.

Not only are chromosome defects common in eggs, sperm, and embryos, but the genetic flaw may prevent the embryo from developing and adjusting to the uterine environment, explaining in part the high rate of embryo loss before implantation. In addition, after embryos become implanted and the pregnancy is recognized, 12 to 15 percent spontaneously abort.

As described earlier in this chapter, when a gene is altered or missing, the result usually is a biochemical disorder leading to illness or mental retardation and, frequently, early death. When the chromosome itself is affected, the baby often is born with defects that can range from mild to severe. If a large segment of the chromosome is abnormal, it usually means that more than one gene is involved and the baby is likely to have multiple defects.

Chromosome defects include too many or too few chromosomes, as well as chromosomes that are flawed because the end sections of two of them changed places, usually at the time of conception. Parts of chromosomes can break off and disappear or become reattached upside down. The pair of chromosomes that determines the sex of the embryo appears to be more susceptible to damage than the other 22 pairs; aberrations in the sex chromosomes may affect intellectual development and function.

Diagnosing Genetic Diseases in Embryos

A procedure for examining the genes of an embryo has been developed. Investigators in England reported early in 1989 that they had removed single cells from 30 three-day-old embryos and had successfully tested the cells for a gene sequence found only on the male-determining Y chromosome. The research demonstrated that it was possible to diagnose genetic diseases in embryos, and it is expected that the test for gender will be useful to women who carry the genes for male-linked diseases such as Duchenne muscular dystrophy, hemophilia, and Lesch-Nyhan syndrome. The test results were confirmed by conventional chromosome testing techniques, which are slower and generally require more genetic material.

To find the gender-determining gene sequence in the cell of the embryo, Dr. Alan H. Handyside, of Hammersmith Hospital in London, and his colleagues used the new, highly sensitive, rapid technique called polymerase chain reaction (PCR) for amplifying gene sequences. PCR has been used on adult cells to identify gene sequences responsible for certain inherited diseases. As PCR tests are developed for specific genetic mutations, scientists believe they could also be used to examine embryos for the diseases. The British group, in fact, has begun to use PCR methodology to test embryos for cystic fibrosis and Duchenne muscular dystrophy.

Current practice with in vitro fertilization indicates that the human embryo develops naturally, even if one or more cells are lost at the eight-cell stage. For this reason, Dr. Handyside believes that removing just one cell will not cause any specific defects if embryos analyzed this way are returned to the mother and developed into fetuses. Dr. Handyside and Professor Robert Winston have received ethical approval from British authorities to transfer tested embryos to their mothers. Clinical trials are already in the early stages; if pregnancies result, chorionic villus sampling will be used to confirm the accuracy of the embryo analyses.

If further research enables scientists to develop tests that can detect both chromosomal abnormalities and gene defects in embryos, it will be possible to choose only healthy embryos for transfer to the uterus during in vitro fertilization. Moreover, couples at risk for giving birth to a child with a hereditary disease could use embryo testing and in vitro fertilization as a way to have a healthy baby—a more desirable alternative to becoming pregnant, testing the fetus, and facing the prospect of having an abortion if the fetus inherited the disease. Observers believe research on embryos is likely to lead to more wanted and healthy children and to a reduction in the number of abortions.

Preserving Embryos by Freezing

For ethical reasons research on normal reproductive processes in laboratory and farm animals has been more acceptable than in human beings, and such widely used procedures as artificial insemination and in vitro fertilization were first performed in animal husbandry. Similarly, the freezing of animal embryos has been carried out successfully since the early 1970s, and today scientists are continuing their attempt to achieve the same good results with the human embryo. The Office of Technology Assessment (OTA) found that about 60 children have been born after frozen and thawed embryos were transferred to their mothers' wombs.

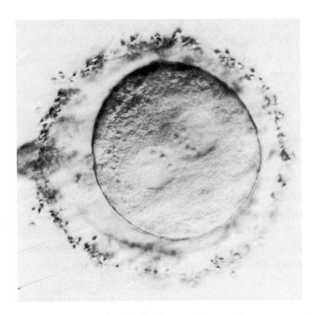

This embryo was frozen shortly after fertilization, at the two-cell stage, as part of an in vitro fertilization treatment for infertility. Implanted in the uterus of its mother months later, it developed into a healthy infant. Credit: Genetics & IVF Institute/Fairfax Cryobank

There are several reasons why preserving human embryos is desirable. In IVF treatment most or all of the eggs retrieved after ovulatory stimulation might be fertilized. To transfer them all to the mother's uterus could result in a multiple pregnancy, which often is hazardous to the mother as well as to the fetuses. Research has demonstrated that embryos not transferred to the uterus during in vitro fertilization can be preserved by freezing and storing, ready to be used if the first embryo transfer is not successful.

Cryopreservation makes it possible to use fewer embryos per transfer and to transfer embryos during a reproductive cycle that has not been stimulated by drugs. Some researchers believe stimulatory drugs may make the uterus less receptive to the implanting embryo. Cryopreservation also substantially reduces the number of retrieval procedures, which means a reduction in cost and patient time.

Approximately half the patients having IVF treatment have their extra embryos frozen. Research at the Genetics & IVF Institute and Fairfax Hospital, in Fairfax, Virginia, found little difference in ability to grow between frozen and thawed embryos and fresh early embryos from the same mother. Almost all (92.7 percent) of the frozen embryos were morphologically intact after thawing and 81.6 percent of them divided, compared to 89.4 percent of the fresh zygotes. The pregnancy rates achieved with the two groups of sibling embryos were also similar.

Improving Embryo Development

Most of the culture media used to nourish eggs and embryos in IVF centers are based on media developed for mouse eggs. If there are significant differences in metabolism between a human egg and a mouse egg, a culture medium tailored more closely to the needs of the human ovum might improve the results of in vitro fertilization.

The metabolic characteristics of the human egg can indicate what enzyme levels it requires in order to survive and develop into an embryo. Oliver H. Lowry and his colleagues at Washington University have developed a method for analyzing a single human egg for its enzymes and metabolites. Their research uncovered enormous differences in enzyme levels between human eggs and mouse eggs. Certain enzyme levels were consistently higher in the human ovum than in the mouse ovum, indicating that the human egg has a greater capacity to burn lipids.

The St. Louis scientists note that the capacity to measure several metabolites and enzymes on the same specimen also may offer opportunities beyond that of describing the normal constitution and energy metabolism of the human egg. The noninvasive test they designed, they note, may provide a way to pinpoint the cause of developmental failures in the eggs themselves, rather than in the culture medium or culture conditions.

The Embryo Research Vacuum

Because there is no public forum for discussing the ethical concerns that surround research on reproduction, very little basic clinical research on human eggs and preimplantation embryos is being carried out in the United States. Without first undergoing consideration by this forum—the defunct Ethics Advisory Board (EAB)—such basic research and clinical studies cannot be funded by the federal government. When the OTA researched its report on infertility, it learned that the National Institutes of Health expected to receive over 100 grant applications for reproductive research if the EAB were ever revived.

Current research on sperm, eggs, and preimplantation embryos uses specimens discarded from infertility programs. As a result, it is not known whether information based on such material will hold true for sperm and eggs produced by couples who do not have fertility problems. Also not known is the effect on human eggs and sperm of environmental influences, such as infection, drugs, radiation, and toxins.

There are two sources of embryos for research: those produced in the laboratory from eggs and sperm donated for research and unused embryos that remain after a successful IVF procedure. Only in Great Britain are both types permitted for study; other countries allow research only with post-IVF embryos. In the United States no laws or federal regulations specifically prohibit research on post-IVF embryos. However, the unsettled nature of the question of federal support for embryo research creates among scientists an uncertainty and reluctance to proceed. Research is limited to observations or measurements rather than interventions.

Until the ethical concerns about such studies are addressed in the United States and guidelines developed, there will be no federally funded, organized program for basic embryo research. For carriers of genetic diseases who want to have children and for infertile couples for whom IVF treatment fails, the lack of a policy regarding embryo research means a substantial delay in medicine's ability to help them have healthy children.

John Fletcher, of the University of Virginia, has said that the absence of federal support for research on reproduction means the scientific basis for the practice of reproductive medicine and medical genetics "is stunted." Dr. Fletcher also noted that:

> Genetic disorders account for one-third of all admissions to pediatric units in hospitals and for almost one-fourth of neonatal mortality. . . . If the pre-embryo is diagnosable, not only couples undergoing infertility treatment could avoid harm to their families and future by embryo diagnosis and selection, but families at higher genetic risk could choose this early form of diagnosis and avoid the emotional and moral suffering of abortion of a wanted pregnancy.

CONCLUSION

Technology makes it increasingly possible to test adults, newborns, and fetuses for genetic diseases. The tests use a variety of approaches, the most recent being the procedures that survey DNA to locate genetic flaws known to account for inherited disorders. Furthermore, research makes it clear that it is possible to detect chromosome abnormalities and genetic errors in the human egg and embryo, making it feasible to implant only healthy embryos during in vitro fertilization. In the future, U.S. couples at risk for having a child with a hereditary disease could be offered embryo testing and in vitro fertilization as a way to have a healthy child.

In another approach toward solving infertility problems, researchers are finding that important aspects of reproductive functioning are governed by the brain. The hypothalamus appears to control the action of the several hormone systems that regulate sperm production and ovulation. Increased understanding of this delicately balanced system has made possible a new treatment for the absence of ovulation, a common cause of female infertility. Further research may identify a relationship among patterns of hormone production and a normal sperm count.

These are important studies, and their results hold the promise of improving the reproductive outcomes of many families. However, a de facto moratorium on federal funding of any research involving fertilized eggs and early embryos cannot be overlooked. It has slowed scientific progress toward a better understanding of normal human reproductive functioning and toward developing procedures that would help couples have healthy children.

ACKNOWLEDGMENTS

This chapter is partially based on presentations by Ernst Knobil, C. Thomas Caskey, Neal First, and John Fletcher.

REFERENCES

Role of the Brain in Reproduction

Fries, H., S.J. Nillius, and F. Pettersson. 1974. Epidemiology of secondary amenorrhea: II. A retrospective evaluation of etiology with special regard to psychogenic factors and weight loss. American Journal of Obstetrics and Gynecology. 15:February:473-479.

Gompel, A., and P. Mauvais-Jarvis. 1988. Induction of ovulation with pulsatile GnRH in hypothalamic amenorrhoea. Human Reproduction. 3(4):473-477.

Knobil, E. 1987. A hypothalamic pulse generator governs mammalian reproduction. News in Physiological Sciences. April:42-43.

Knobil, E. 1988. The neuroendocrine control of ovulation. Human Reproduction. 3(4):469-472.

Marx, J.L. 1988. Sexual responses are—almost—all in the brain. Science. 241:903-904.

Pohl, C.R., and E. Knobil. 1982. The role of the central nervous system in the control of ovarian function in higher primates. Annual Review of Physiology. 44:583-593.

Pettersson, F., H. Fries, and S.J. Nillius. 1973. Epidemiology of secondary amenorrhea: I. Incidence and prevalence rates. American Journal of Obstetrics and Gynecology. Sept. 1:80-86.

Santoro, N., M. Filicori, and W.F. Crowley, Jr. 1986. Hypogonadotropic disorders in men and women: diagnosis and therapy with pulsatile GnRH. Endocrine Review. Vol. 7:11-23.

Santoro, N., M.E. Wierman, M. Filicori, J. Waldstreicher, and W.F. Crowley, Jr. 1986. Intravenous administration of pulsatile gonadotropin-releasing hormone in hypothalamic amenorrhea: effects of dosage. Journal of Clinical Endocrinology and Metabolism. 62(1):109-116.

Diagnosis of Genetic Diseases

Appelman, Z., and M.S. Golbus. 1987. Uses of fetal tissue sampling. Contemporary Ob/Gyn: Special Issue: Update on Surgery. 42-49.

Caskey, C.T. 1987. Disease diagnosis by recombinant DNA methods. Science. 236:1223-1229.

Kolata, G. 1988. Fetuses treated through umbilical cords. New York Times. March 29, C-1.

Kolata, G. 1989. Scientists pinpoint genetic changes that predict cancer. New York Times. May 16, C-1.

"Genetic Series." 1985-1989. Pamphlets produced by the March of Dimes Birth Defects Foundation.

Milunsky, A. 1989. *Choices, Not Chances.* Boston: Little Brown and Company.

Nichols, E. 1988. *Human Gene Therapy.* Institute of Medicine, National Academy of Sciences. Cambridge, MA: Harvard University Press.

The New Human Genetics: How Gene Splicing Helps Researchers Fight Inherited Disease. 1984. Written by Maya Pines. Bethesda, MD: National Institute of General Medical Sciences, National Institutes of Health. NIH Publication 84-662.

Rhoads, G.G., et al. 1989. The safety and efficacy of chorionic villus sampling for early prenatal diagnosis of cytogenetic abnormalities. New England Journal of Medicine. 320:609-617.

Thomas, P. 1988. Fetuses treated by cordocentesis. Medical World News. June 13, 95-96.

Research on Embryo Health

Chi, M.M., J. Manchester, V.C. Yang, A.D. Curato, R.C. Strickler, and O.H. Lowry. 1988. Contrast in levels of metabolic enzymes in human and mouse ova. Biology of Reproduction. 39:295-307.

Fletcher, J.C. 1989. How abortion politics stifle science. The Washington Post. February 5, D-3.

Fugger, E.F., M. Bustells, L.P. Katz, A.D. Dorfman, S.D. Bender, and J.D. Schulman. 1988. Embryonic development and pregnancy from fresh and cryopreserved sibling pronucleate human zygotes. Fertility and Sterility. 50(2):273-277.

Martin, R.H., M.M. Mahadevan, P.J. Taylor, K. Hildebrand, L. Long-Simpson, D. Peterson, J. Yamamoto, and J. Fleetham. 1986. Chromosomal analysis of unfertilized human oocytes. Journal of Reproductive Fertility. 78:673-678.

McLaren, A. 1988. The IVF conceptus: research today and tomorrow. In *In Vitro Fertilization and Other Assisted Reproduction*. Edited by H.W. Jones and C. Schrader. Annals of the New York Academy of Sciences. 541:639-645.

McLaughlin, L. 1982. *The Pill, John Rock, and the Church*. Boston: Little Brown and Co.

Office of Technology Assessment. *Infertility: Medical and Social Choices*. 1988. Washington, D.C.: U.S. Congress, OTA-BA-358.

Plachot, M., et al. 1988. Chromosomal analysis of human oocytes and embryos in an in vitro fertilization program. In *In Vitro Fertilization and Other Assisted Reproduction*. Edited by H.W. Jones and C. Schrader. Annals of the New York Academy of Sciences. 541:384-397.

Wallach, E.E. 1988. Hail to the animal kingdom. Fertility and Sterility. 50(4):552-554.

Weiss, R. 1989. Test screens live "test tube" embryos. Science News, March 4, 135:132.

Wood, E.C. 1988. The future of in vetro fertilization. In *In Vitro Fertilization and Other Assisted Reproduction*. Edited by H.W. Jones and C. Schrader. Annals of the New York Academy of Sciences. 541:715-721.

Wramsby, H., K. Fredga, and P. Liedholm. 1987. Chromosome analysis of human oocytes recovered from preovulatory follicles in stimulated cycles. New England Journal of Medicine. 316(3):121-124.

7
New Technologies
The Ethical and Social Issues

Research relating to new technologies in the field of reproductive health is important for many reasons, particularly because such research concerns the creation of the next generation and because the methods being applied represent a marked break with tradition. Artificial insemination, in vitro fertilization, and the manipulation of embryos have greatly changed what was once the private province of two people joined in a socially approved union. Professor Patricia A. King, of Georgetown University Law Center, has said that the new reproductive technologies are controversial:

> because they challenge deeply held moral, ethical, and religious values, particularly those values that concern the family and relationships among its members. They involve the deliberate separation of reproduction from the act of human sexuality and from the human body.

Important ethical questions also attend many of the social aspects of reproductive health, such as the issues of hospitals turning away women in labor because they do not have insurance or of routine four-week waits before women can begin prenatal care.

When in vitro fertilization was being discussed in the the early 1970s, some theologians and other critics in the United States and other countries attacked the procedure as representing unethical experimentation on human beings. The chief moral argument against the fertilization of a human egg in a laboratory dish was that the parents' desire for a child did not entitle them to have it by a possibly unsafe method that might result in a deformed infant.

In the United States that argument delayed the further development of IVF. In England, where the perspective on moral issues was somewhat different, Drs. Patrick Steptoe and Robert Edwards continued their research and in 1978 achieved a successful live birth by IVF. In the years since, thousands of infants have been born worldwide as the result of IVF. As experience with the technique accumulates, the risk to the embryo is clearly no greater than it is in nature, nor are the parents at any increased risk of harm. The ethical concerns about the safety of the technique have largely subsided. Dr. Kenneth Ryan says:

> Although similar questions of safety will be raised for any new reproductive technology that is developed, such as cryopreservation of embryos and ova, the moral roadblock to taking risk for the unborn has for the time being been breached.

Today ethical questions regarding reproductive technology are not focused so much on the safety of the technology itself but on how it is applied and on where it might be leading. The future of IVF will depend on whether research is allowed and what types of studies are permitted. In the 1980s the major question for this technology was whether it was morally right to create life in a dish. In the 1990s, as scientists become increasingly able to analyze (and perhaps alter) the DNA of an embryo, ethical questions will focus on what, if any, limits should be set for embryo manipulation.

Basic research on IVF and embryo development would add considerably to the information base affecting all of reproductive health. Such work would increase physician understanding of the fundamentals of reproduction, of normal pregnancy and normal fetal growth, of the causes of premature labor, and of the reproductive system's marked susceptibility to cancer. It would assist research for safer, more effective birth control. The disbanding of the Ethics Advisory Board (EAB) not only blocked research on IVF and embryo development, but it also slowed progress on the study of reproduction.

The ability of scientists to sustain human embryos in the laboratory for a week or longer has opened up enormous possibilities in terms of what could be done with sperm, eggs, and the early human embryo. This technology raises questions about our obligations as a society to these gametes and early embryos and about the ethical basis for these obligations. These questions will need to be resolved in order for research on reproductive health to be federally funded and to move forward. As Professor David T. Ozar, of Loyola University, and other observers have noted, "A nation cannot resolve by law and public policy a set of issues on which there is not, within the community at large, a consensus on the underlying values."

EARLY DEVELOPMENT OF THE EMBRYO

Although research on human embryos has been severely limited by a lack of federal support, studies of animals have contributed to scientists' understanding of many aspects of reproduction. Privately funded investigations have focused on what happens at specific points in the development of a human egg into an embryo. An understanding of this process is imperative to the formation of sound ethical arguments about infertility treatments and basic research on the human embryo.

The egg and sperm are haploid cells, cells that contain only half their full complement of chromosomes. After the egg is fertilized by a sperm, a complex series of chromosomal changes occur that ultimately result in a blending of the DNA from the sperm with the DNA of the egg to form a single cell, or zygote, that contains the full complement of chromosomes.

From this single cell, all the tissues and organs of the human being, as well as surrounding tissues, such as the placenta, will develop. Cell division occurs several times, forming a tiny cluster of 12 to 16 cells, or the morula. The morula develops a fluid-filled inner cavity as it moves slowly through the fallopian tube. By the time the cluster reaches the uterus, three to four days after fertilization, the cells that will become the embryo can be distinguished from the cells that will form the placenta and fetal membranes. At this stage the cell cluster is termed a blastocyst.

The blastocyst develops a covering of cells that enable it to bind to the surface of the uterus. The uterine lining is receptive to the blastocyst for only a short time after ovulation. If the blastocyst implants successfully, on about the 11th day after fertilization the cells begin to differentiate into layers that are precursors of different tissues, although at this time the inner cell mass can still divide and develop into two separate individuals.

After the 18th day, the basic patterns of the organ systems, including the nervous system, begin to develop. The process continues, and after the ninth week, development advances to the point that the embryo is defined as a fetus. The fetal stage lasts until birth. During this period the organ systems develop further and the fetus matures and grows in size.

As noted in Chapter 6, during fertilization and the first stages of cell division, the chance of a chromosomal mishap is substantial. Pioneering studies by Arthur Hertig and John Rock at Harvard showed that one-third to two-thirds of eggs and approximately 25 percent of embryos have abnormal chromosomes. For this reason and others not yet fully understood, the vast majority of human embryos do not develop as far as the blastocyst stage.

Furthermore, if the uterus and blastocyst have not been adequately primed by the production of certain key hormones, implantation may not occur. A substantial proportion of early embryos do not implant and simply disappear, probably flushed from the uterus during menstruation. For the early human embryo, developmental failure appears to be the norm.

THE NEED FOR MORE RESEARCH

Although very sophisticated techniques are in use at IVF clinics, the success rates for IVF remain low. Because reproductive research is funded chiefly by major IVF centers, pharmaceutical companies, and universities, it has been sparse, uneven, and without established priorities. As a result, there are considerable gaps in our knowledge of the reproductive process and embryo development. Moreover, as mentioned in earlier chapters, the absence of federal support means no federal oversight of this research because the National Institutes of Health does not provide scientific peer review for private research.

A better understanding of the basics of reproduction and embryo development not only has the potential for improving infertility treatments, but it also is expected to contribute to many aspects of reproductive health. A recent Institute of Medicine study noted the existence of substantial deficiencies in the scientific underpinnings of reproductive biology. The study also pinpointed many areas in which further research could contribute to the improvement of infertility treatments.

The study noted that these deficiencies occur in the basic sciences that underlie the techniques used in various infertility treatments and in embryo transfer. Scientific knowledge that leads to improved infertility therapies may also be applied to the development of better contraceptive technologies. The study identified over 40 areas that need further research.

Some of the research questions that remain unanswered are:

- How do we identify a viable embryo?
- How does cryopreservation affect sperm, eggs, and embryos?
- What is the optimum number of embryos to transfer during IVF?
- Why does development stop in some embryos after a normal beginning?
- What are the physiological effects of hormone treatments?
- What factors control egg maturation and what factors control implantation?
- What are the elements that lead to the natural wastage of eggs and embryos and how do they operate?

One area just beginning to be studied is the diagnosis of genetic and chromosomal disorders in the early embryo before it is transferred to the uterus, as described in Chapter 6. John Fletcher estimates that genetic disorders account for one-third of all admissions to pediatric units and for almost 25 percent of neonatal mortality. The optimal goal of diagnosing inherited diseases in the early embryo, he believes, would be the ability to analyze sperm and eggs, so fertilization could be achieved with gametes that do not carry harmful genes.

Aside from studies on infertility, the 10-year de facto moratorium on reproductive health research has dampened studies that could improve the health of mothers and infants. Some examples:

- Little is known about normal pregnancy and normal fetal development and what can occur during this process to cause nongenetic diseases or birth defects.
- Factors that lead to premature labor have yet to be identified.
- More information is needed about the unusual vulnerability of the reproductive system to malignancies.
- Additional knowledge might make it possible to ease the heavy drain of pregnancy on the body.
- More insight into the endocrine control of ovulation that occurs during breastfeeding might aid in the spacing of births.
- Most male infertility is of unknown origin; research is needed to uncover the causes.

ETHICAL AND SOCIAL CONCERNS

Certain ethical or social issues aroused by some approaches to infertility treatment and by embryo research focus on research in these areas;

other issues are concerned with aspects of the clinical practice. The latter include concerns about the safety of donated sperm, the confidentiality of sperm donors, and the right of a child born as the result of donor sperm to know his or her complete parentage or the genetic/medical aspects of that parentage. Questions have also been raised about the moral and legal status of early embryos and the fate of those that are not used in IVF treatment, including frozen embryos. Equally basic are questions regarding the right of an individual to reproduce; the sale of embryos, eggs, and sperm; and the pros and cons of defining infertility as a disease, which would affect insurance coverage.

Ethical concerns that have a direct bearing on research can have important consequences on the funding for that research. The moral status given the embryo in each stage of its development will dictate what research or manipulation is considered acceptable at that stage. Such issues as the disposal of unneeded embryos, the creation of embryos expressly for research, and the point at which embryo development research should be permitted are strongly affected by how society perceives the embryo.

Not surprisingly, analyses of the ethical stances taken by various segments of society reveal a range of positions concerning embryo research. At one end of the spectrum is the Roman Catholic Church and other religious groups that believe life begins when the two haploid cells, the egg and the sperm, unite to form a chromosomally complete cell. The Vatican's *Instruction on Respect for Human Life in Its Origin and on the Dignity of Procreation,* issued in 1987, declares that no moral distinction can be made among any stages of the embryo. According to this position, the absolute sanctity accorded to human life begins with the fertilized egg, making it impossible to discard early embryos or to use them for research.

At the other end of the spectrum are those who contend that an embryo is simply a group of living cells and that any value attached to this biological material is in the eye of the beholder. Those who hold this view often point out that a large proportion of naturally conceived embryos do not develop after implantation and that discarding human embryos can be viewed as a similar process.

Between these two views lie the positions taken by a number of nations that have systematically examined the issues relating to the new reproductive technologies.

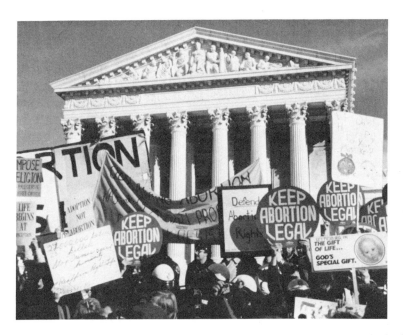

Both sides of the abortion issue demonstrate outside the Supreme Court in April 1989. Credit: Uniphoto/Paul Conklin

RESOLVING ETHICAL AND SOCIAL CONCERNS

Since the mid-1970s countries in which the new reproductive technologies are in use have relied on public discussion to resolve the ethical and social issues that arise. A national public committee is appointed to analyze the issues and to formulate a public policy. The committee, in turn, often receives testimony from technical experts, laypersons, and other committees representing various interest groups. It is a public process of give and take with the goal of achieving a consensus. The officially appointed group then seeks to reach ethical judgments that are both rationally defensible and politically acceptable to large segments of its society. To do so, it often seeks the middle ground on an issue.

LeRoy Walters, Director of Bioethics at the Kennedy Institute of Ethics at Georgetown University, has analyzed the statements formulated by these committees. For example, four Australian committees found research on preimplantation embryos ethically unacceptable. Commissions in other countries approved of some kinds of early embryo research, with 6 of 11 accepting research only on embryos left over from treatment programs. Five committee statements, including one from the 1979 U.S.

EAB, allowed the creation of embryos through IVF for research purposes. The majority of the committees agreed that no research should be
permitted on embryos after 14 days following laboratory fertilization.

Many of the recommendations made by these committees have been
written into laws controlling certain aspects of infertility therapies or the
research associated with them, or both. Dr. Walters observes:

> Committee statements represent a substantial contribution to the bio-
> ethics literature on the new reproductive technologies. One can, in fact,
> trace a kind of evolution in international ethical reflection on these technolo-
> gies.

Although Dr. Walters says that committees, commissions, and boards
are not likely to replace the work of legislatures, government agencies,
and the courts, he feels that periodic committee statements and reports
may become the preferred mode of public oversight and social control
for at least certain areas of biology and medicine.

A similar approach was attempted in the United States in the late
1970s when the EAB was formed. Research involving IVF presented
ethical problems for the federal government because religious and right-
to-life groups opposed a technique that sometimes results in the destruc-
tion of fertilized eggs. The EAB was established in 1978 to review all
proposals for federal funds for research on reproduction for the U.S.
Department of Health and Human Services (DHHS). In 1979 the EAB
made a favorable recommendation for federal support of embryo research
to evaluate IVF safety and efficacy. In 1980 the EAB was disbanded.
Since then there has been no official body to carry out the department's
regulations regarding research on IVF and other aspects of reproduction
or to review proposals for scientific studies in this field.

The lack of an official avenue for requesting federal funds for such
research has had two effects: The development of new knowledge about
reproduction, normal pregnancy and fetal development, and the human
embryo has either slowed markedly or is not being performed. Whatever
research exists is financed privately. Although in July 1988 the DHHS
announced plans to recharter the EAB, this has not happened.

Meanwhile, the two professional societies in the United States that
represent the physicians most involved with IVF have given careful consideration to the ethical issues arising from IVF and associated embryo
research. The ethics committee of the American College of Obstetricians and Gynecologists (ACOG) in 1986 outlined a set of standards
to guide research on early embryos. The ACOG recommended using

human embryos only when nonhuman embryos could not provide the needed information and studying embryos only up to the 14th day of development.

The American Fertility Society (AFS) also examined the ethics of infertility treatment and research. The AFS listed eight technologies that it felt were ethically acceptable, including IVF and embryo transfer, the use of donor eggs, and the use of frozen donor sperm. Six procedures, including the use of frozen eggs and studies of early embryos before the 14th day of development, were viewed as suitable for clinical experimentation. A year later, after reviewing the Vatican's newly issued *Instruction on Respect for Human Life*, the AFS responded in summary that progressive degrees of respect for the human embryo should accompany its progressive development and that experimentation on embryos can be justified and is necessary if the human condition is to be improved.

In 1985 a congressional Biomedical Ethics Board was created. To be comprised of six senators and six representatives, the board was assigned to look into the protection of human subjects in federally funded biomedical research. The selection of members and a 14-member advisory committee of scientists, physicians, clergy, and others became an extremely laborious process. Disagreements, chiefly about the prospective appointees' views on abortion and other ethical questions, such as the definition of human life, considerably slowed the formation of the advisory committee. In late 1989 the board ceased to function because of a political impasse over abortion.

CONCLUSION

Research on new reproductive technologies challenges many of the deeply held moral, ethical, and religious values of society, particularly because such technologies include the separation of reproduction from the act of human union and from the body. Although ethical concerns about the safety of these methods have ebbed, society is now concerned about how the technologies are applied and where they might be leading. The ability to sustain human embryos in the laboratory and, in coming years, the increasing ability to analyze and manipulate them raise questions about what obligations society has to such embryos.

Enough is known about early embryo development to realize that it is a multistage process and that a large proportion of embryos are flawed and fail to implant in the uterus. An understanding of embryo development is important in order to form sound ethical judgments about infertility therapies and embryo research. Although the techniques used for IVF are sophisticated, the success rates for the procedure remain low, and there is still a lot to be learned about the reproductive process and about embryos.

Since the EAB was discontinued in 1980, studies have been few and privately funded. The congressional Biomedical Ethics Board, formed in 1985 to examine on a broad scale the issues associated with the use of human subjects in reproductive research, is nonfunctional. As noted earlier, without a federal policy and without federal funding, there is no organized direction or peer review. Also, studies aimed at improving maternal and fetal health and women's reproductive health in general are impeded by the absence of an ethics review body.

More important, without an active ethics review board there is no public mechanism for addressing the ethical and social concerns that research on reproductive health can arouse. These concerns are many, and the ethical positions on each can be wide ranging. In other nations, appointed committees have successfully achieved a public concensus. Their recommendations have been written into laws to control ethically sensitive aspects of infertility treatments and embryo research. Scientists, ethicists, and other observers have strongly urged that the United States follow a similar course. They suggest reviving the EAB in order to resolve ethical and social concerns about reproductive technology in this country. An active EAB would make it possible to plan the basic research necessary to improve such technology.

ACKNOWLEDGMENT

Chapter 7 is based in part on presentations made by Kenneth Ryan, John Fletcher, and Patricia King.

REFERENCES

American College of Obstetricians and Gynecologists. 1984. Human In Vitro Fertil-ization and Embryo Placement. Committee on Gynecologic Practice. Committee Statement. Washington, D.C.

American College of Obstetricians and Gynecologists. 1986. Ethical Issues in Human In Vitro Fertilization and Embryo Placement. Committee on Ethics, ACOG Committee Opinion Number 47. Washington, D.C.

Andrews, L.B. 1987. Ethical and legal aspects of in vitro fertilization and artifical insemination by donor. Urologic Clinics of North America. 14(3):633-642.

Elias, S., and G.J. Annas. 1986. Social policy considerations in noncoital reproduction. Journal of the American Medical Association. 255(1):62-68.

Fertility and Sterility. 1988b. Ethical considerations of the new reproductive technologies. By the Ethics Committee (1986-7) of the American Fertility Society, in light of Instruction on the Respect for Human Life in Its Origin and on the Dignity of Procreation, issued by the Congregation for the Doctrine of the Faith. Vol. 49, Supplement 1.

Fletcher, J.C. 1989. How abortion politics stifle science. The Washington Post. February 5, D-3.

Institute of Medicine. 1989. *Medically Assisted Conception: An Agenda for Research.* Washington, D.C.: National Academy Press.

King, P.A. 1986. Reproductive technologies. In the looseleaf series, *BioLaw.* Frederick, MD: University Publications of America.

Norman, C. 1988. IVF research moratorium to end? Science. 241:405-406.

Ozar, D.T. 1985. The case against thawing unused frozen embryos. Hastings Center Report, August, 7-12.

Ryan, K.J. 1989. The ethics of current reproductive technologies. In *Problems in Reproductive Endocrinology and Infertility.* Edited by Michael R. Soules. New York: Elsevier Science Publishing Company, Inc.

Walters, L. 1985. Ethical issues in human in vitro fertilization and embryo transfer. In *Genetics and the Law III.* Edited by A. Milunsky and G.J. Annas. New York: Plenum Press.

Walters, L. 1987. Ethics and new reproductive technologies: an international review of committee statements. Hastings Center Report, Special Supplement, June.

Wood, E.C. 1988. The future of in vitro fertilization. In *In Vitro Fertilization and Other Assisted Reproduction.* Edited by H.W. Jones and C. Schrader. Annals of the New York Academy of Sciences. 541:715-721.

8

Areas for Policy Development

At the Institute of Medicine (IOM) annual meeting from which this volume was developed, a panel of specialists examined the issues in reproductive health that they considered to be of the greatest concern. The importance of reproductive health as an indicator of the overall well-being and vigor of the nation was emphasized. The speakers and many of those in attendance discussed recent scientific advances and the unresolved social issues of reproductive biology. These two points became clear:

- As a nation it appears we have not decided whether our goal is to control the sexual activity of our teenagers or to devote our resources to improving reproductive health and decreasing the number of unplanned and unwanted pregnancies.
- As a heterogeneous people, our concerns are diverse. Without a public body to consider all points of view in the emotionally charged realm of sexuality and reproduction and to develop a factual and analytic basis for enlightened public policy making, it is extremely difficult for a nation to formulate policy.

Although a number of issues concerning reproductive health have been resolved, new ones materialize as society evolves and more is learned about reproduction and the importance of improving the health

158

of mothers and babies. Worldwide the emergence of new technologies has prompted vigorous discussions of their social and ethical aspects. In the United States the task of developing a consensus on reproductive health issues has proved much more difficult, partly because of this country's diversity and its unwillingness to discuss sexually related issues frankly. Commissions and boards have been mandated, but conflicting opinions and a reluctance to become involved in such controversial issues made even the process of appointing members difficult. Without the sustained, active interest of the nation's leaders to support them, no board has survived long enough either to resolve ethical questions about individual research projects or to establish a broad consensus about the ethical issues that arise from such research. As a result, major needs affecting reproductive health are not being met:

• *The need for federal support of research on the reproductive system.*

Information from studies that use human eggs and embryos would be more reliable and of better quality if the research received the direction and organization that accompany most federally supported projects. The public is excluded from participating in the evaluation of research in which it has displayed a keen interest. The absence of an Ethics Advisory Board (EAB) has halted reproductive health investigations that hold promise. Moreover, infertile people and families at high risk for genetic diseases are being deprived of the potential benefits of research.

• *Standards, licensing, and government regulation are needed for IVF clinics.*

In vitro fertilization and gamete intrafallopian transfer techniques have moved rapidly from experimental to therapeutic status without benefit of federal oversight. Although professional societies have set minimum standards for the new infertility treatments, clinics are not obliged to adhere to them. In addition, embryo laboratories are not licensed. Before the Wyden subcommittee surveyed IVF clinics, information on their number, services, and success rates was limited. At present, users of the new infertility treatments have little protection under the law.

• *Strategies to prevent infertility should be developed and widely promoted.*

Because infertility can be emotionally devastating and expensive to treat, reducing its incidence is desirable. In some 20 percent of infertile

U.S. couples, the disorder was caused by infectious disease, a type of infertility that is preventable. Many cases of infertility are caused by fallopian tube obstructions resulting from repeated bouts of sexually transmitted diseases. A massive national effort is needed to educate public health professionals as well as the public about the relationship between sexually transmitted diseases and infertility, the symptoms of these diseases, and the optimal treatments. The effort should incorporate partner tracing and patient counseling.

• *The nation's maternity care system needs to be reorganized and improved.*

The United States in recent years has not been able to achieve a real decrease in its neonatal mortality rate. In addition, it is experiencing a deepening of poverty, particularly among single mothers, and there appears to be no change in the rate of births to teenagers and unmarried women, who often have low birthweight babies. Prenatal care is clearly associated with improved pregnancy outcomes. It reduces the incidence of maternal and infant deaths and low birthweight among newborns. Prenatal care is especially important for women who are at increased medical or social risk, or both. Women who do not receive adequate maternity care have double the risk of having a low birthweight infant.

Prenatal care is also cost-effective. Researchers estimate that every dollar spent on prenatal care for women who risk having a low birthweight baby potentially reduces by over $3 the cost for medical care for that baby during its first year.

Since 1980 the percentage of women who received late or no prenatal care has increased. Although this trend applies to all races, the increase is most notable among black women. An IOM study revealed maternity care to be a complicated network of publicly and privately funded services that is "flawed, fragmented, and overly complex." According to the IOM report, the best way to reverse current declines in the use of prenatal care would be a complete transformation of the present nonsystem. The IOM committee strongly denounced the present practice of making incremental changes to existing services.

It emphasized the importance of making no alterations in the maternity care system "until the nation's leaders first make a commitment to enact substantial changes." In addition, it recommended that improvements to the maternity care system be accompanied by a greater investment in family planning.

- *A deeper national commitment to family planning education and services is needed.*

The high rates of abortion and teenage pregnancy in the United States indicate the need for more accessible, user-oriented family planning services and education. Many men and women, particularly younger ones, are badly informed about birth control and about the true effectiveness and health risks of the currently available contraceptive methods. To reduce the number of abortions and unintended pregnancies, this country needs to develop a more positive, less equivocal attitude toward contraception and needs to acknowledge in a variety of forums the importance of family planning to good reproductive health. Accompanying a more open attitude toward contraception should be a vigorous advertising and public education campaign about family planning and birth control. In addition, ways should be found to ameliorate the current impediments to contraceptive research and development.

- *Better researched programs are needed if adolescents are going to be helped successfully to avoid pregnancy or to delay sexual activity.*

Although sexual activity among U.S. teenagers is no more prevalent than among adolescents in other industrialized countries, the United States has much higher rates of adolescent childbearing and abortion. In recent years many programs have tried to reduce the incidence of teen pregnancy, but their results are not clear. A much better understanding of what program elements are most effective in helping teens avoid sexual activity and pregnancy is necessary. To achieve this, the IOM committee on prenatal care suggested that programs using new approaches should include a research component designed to demonstrate what did and did not work in that program.

- *A public policy process is needed.*

None of the above issues can be resolved without a public policy process. During the 1970s medical researchers learned to create human life in a dish—to fertilize the human egg and nurture the resulting embryo through its first stages of development. The 1990s will see an expansion of technological skills for analyzing the embryo, enabling scientists to recognize abnormal chromosomes and to detect genes known to produce physical diseases and, perhaps, genes suspected of producing mental disorders or antisocial behaviors.

The ethical implications of such expertise, which already exists and is being expanded in other countries and, with private support, in the United States, are enormous. Because of its nature, this research should be done with federal input and controls, and both the support and controls should reflect the concerns of this society. As other countries have demonstrated, a national public commission or board is an effective tool for analyzing broad ethical issues and for formulating public policy. Using this approach, nations have successfully developed laws governing ethically sensitive research and have established criteria for licensing specific research projects.

The United States possessed such a public entity in the congressional Biomedical Ethics Board, formed in 1985 to examine the protection of human subjects in biomedical research. The board ceased to function in 1989.

The United States would have the equivalent of a licensing body in the Ethics Advisory Board if the U.S. Department of Health and Human Services moves on its proposal to reactivate it. Like the Biomedical Ethics Board, the EAB also had a politically difficult task; it was allowed to lapse in 1980 when its funding and charter expired.

Meanwhile, privately supported, ethically sensitive research is being carried out in the United States without federal oversight, and therapies for infertility are being developed and used without the safeguard of a solid scientific basis. The success of infertility treatments has been limited partially because the scientific knowledge on which they are based is insufficient.

The genetic testing of early embryos holds the promise of drastically reducing the use of later abortions for severe birth defects. Such tests would also make it possible for families with a history of genetic disease to have healthy babies. Without a means for resolving the ethical issues associated with embryo research, however, these lines of study cannot be explored under federal guidelines.

In order to give the public a voice in and some control over the ethically sensitive issues associated with reproduction research and treatments, a process of public education on important bioethical issues must be put in place and a national consensus must be developed. Observers have recommended that the EAB be reactivated, energized, and adequately funded. Because the United States is a disparate society, the task of achieving a consensus will be more difficult than it has been for other countries, but these issues must be addressed if the nation is to benefit from reproductive research.

Acknowledgments

The 1988 annual meeting of the Institute of Medicine owes its substance to a number of members, staff, and other experts, but to no one more than the speakers, who also graciously cooperated during the preparation of this book:

KENNETH RYAN (*Chairman*), Kate Macy Ladd Professor of Obstetrics and Gynecology, Harvard Medical School
C. THOMAS CASKEY, Henry and Emma Meyer Professor in Molecular Genetics and Director, Institute for Molecular Genetics, Baylor University College of Medicine
CARL DJERASSI, Professor of Chemistry, Stanford University
ROBERT EDWARDS, Physiological Laboratory, Cambridge University
DANIEL FEDERMAN, Professor of Medicine and Dean for Students and Alumni, Harvard Medical School
NEAL FIRST, Professor of Reproductive Physiology, University of Wisconsin
JOHN FLETCHER, Professor of Biomedical Ethics and of Religious Studies, University of Virginia School of Medicine and College of Arts and Sciences
DEBORAH HENSLER, Director of Research, Institute for Civil Justice, The RAND Corporation
PATRICIA KING, Professor of Law, Georgetown Law Center
LORRAINE KLERMAN, Professor of Public Health, Yale University School of Medicine

ERNST KNOBIL, H. Wayne Hightower Professor and Director, Laboratory for Neuroendocrinology, University of Texas Health Science Center at Houston

MALCOLM POTTS, President, Family Health International

SUSAN SCRIMSHAW, Professor of Public Health and Anthropology and Associate Director, Latin American Center, University of California, Los Angeles

Index

Abortifacients, 43, 66, 91
Abortions, 7
  contraception and, 2, 44, 52–53, 55, 91
  genetic testing and, 132, 134, 135, 162
  health risks of, 91
  rates, 1, 2, 7, 44, 52, 53–54, 62, 69, 70,
    79, 94, 161
  spontaneous, from IVF, 32, 133, 134, 135,
    138
  teenage pregnancy and, 8, 53–54, 62, 69,
    70, 79, 91, 94
Abstinence, 55
Adoption, 14, 87
Adrenal gland dysfunction, 21
Age, and contraceptive use, 76
Agency for International Development, 54
A. H. Robins Company, 45
Aid to Families with Dependent Children, 9,
    81, 87, 113
AIDS, 7, 23
Alan Guttmacher Institute, 43, 52, 60, 61,
    70, 81, 85, 88, 89, 94, 104, 111
Alza Corporation, 45
Amenorrhea, 127, 128
American Academy of Pediatrics, 107, 116
American Association of Tissue Banks, 24,
    28
American Civil Liberties Union, 87

American College of Obstetricians and
    Gynecologists, 28, 47, 107–108, 116,
    154–155
American Fertility Society, 28, 30, 32, 155
American Medical Association Diagnostic
    and Therapeutic Technology
    Assessment panel, 61
Amniocentesis, 134–136
Anencephaly, 135
Anorexia nervosa, 128
Artificial insemination, 3, 5, 11, 12, 23–25,
    26, 28, 140, 147

Basal body temperature, 20
Benign breast tumors, 56
Biodegradable pellets, contraceptive, 65
Biomedical Ethics Board, 155, 156, 162
Birth control, *see* Contraception and
    contraceptives; *and specific methods*
Birth control pills, 2, 57
  availability of, 43, 44, 59, 60, 6, 89–90
  and breast cancer, 55–56, 62
  components, 56
  costs, 46
  development, 41
  effectiveness of, 63
  liability claims, 45–46
  for men, 42

165